'Thanks so much for inviting me to read this heartfelt exploration of your work together, and the transformative potential of the supervision relationship. It has helped to reinforce and significantly extend my sense of what supervision at its best can be about. I am in awe at the way you have translated and explained your experience of relationship so clearly. I am struck by how effectively you have blended your two voices.'

Henry Campion, *MB, BS, Executive Coach Supervisor*

'The hallmarks of this wonderful contribution include the authors' willingness to role-model vulnerability, their compelling commitment to their own learning and that of others – including ours as readers – the intellectual rigour and, of course, the mindfulness, love, and compassion that radiate from the book's pages and underpin their work. These combine in a challenge and invitation to reconsider and deepen our approach to relationships in coaching supervision, coaching and beyond.'

Liz Hall, *editor of* Coaching at Work,
and author of Mindful Coaching

Mindfulness-Based Relational Supervision

Mindfulness-Based Relational Supervision explores a relational and mindfulness-based approach to adult learning and development that is mutually transformational.

The initial focus of the book is a case study that shows the evolution of a dialogical supervision relationship that was transformational for both parties. The authors present their reflections and analysis of key transformational moments that brought insights which significantly enhanced their personal and professional development. The authors adopt an interdisciplinary approach, discussing relational neurobiology and relational mindfulness practice together with ideas from child and adult development, attachment theory, intersubjectivity, somatic experiencing, and adult learning theories. The case study narrative charts the development of the authors' supervision relationship, following which they share a meta-perspective on their learning journey. Finally, they discuss the implications of the study for the education and training of relational practitioners in supervision, coaching, and related fields.

The book will appeal to students, practitioners and supervisors in the helping professions, in particular counselling, psychotherapy, and coaching.

Fiona Adamson is an award-winning Executive Coach Supervisor and author with 40 years' supervision experience. Working with relational mindfulness has transformed her practice through her ability to be present, compassionate, and loving. This creates the conditions for a mutually rich learning experience. She lives in South Hertfordshire with her dear wife Judith.

Jane Brendgen is an Adult Development Coach, Mindfulness Supervisor and founder of Compassionate Cultures, an enterprise focusing on supporting organisations to build compassionate cultures of trust through changing how people relate to one another. Mindfulness and compassion lie at the heart of this work. She lives in a leafy area of Lewes, East Sussex with her Siamese cat Tao.

Mindfulness-Based Relational Supervision

Mutual Learning and Transformation

Fiona Adamson and
Jane Brendgen

Routledge
Taylor & Francis Group
LONDON AND NEW YORK

First published 2022
by Routledge
2 Park Square, Milton Park, Abingdon, Oxon OX14 4RN

and by Routledge
605 Third Avenue, New York, NY 10158

Routledge is an imprint of the Taylor & Francis Group, an informa business

British Library Cataloguing-in-Publication Data
A catalogue record for this book is available from the British Library

Library of Congress Cataloging-in-Publication Data
A catalog record has been requested for this book

ISBN: 978-1-138-06287-0 (hbk)
ISBN: 978-1-138-06310-5 (pbk)
ISBN: 978-1-315-16128-0 (ebk)

DOI: 10.4324/9781315161280

Typeset in Sabon
by Newgen Publishing UK

‘A loving heart is the truest wisdom.’

Charles Dickens, *David Copperfield*

Contents

Acknowledgements

We have been inspired, loved, and helped by many people throughout the writing of this book. We are grateful to Henry Campion for the poem 'The Space Between Us'. He wrote it for us, and we are pleased to include it in our book.

First, we are grateful to Liz Hall, Alison Evans, Emma Donaldson-Feilder, Mark McMordie, Henry Campion, Alison Hodge, and Pam Mclean, who carefully read through our draft manuscript and offered such helpful suggestions. We restructured the book and feel it is a much better read as a result.

We wish to thank and acknowledge the Routledge team that has supported us throughout the process. This includes Joanna Forshaw, Daradi Patar, Lekshmi Priya and Susan Jarvis for her final editing.

Fiona

Jane has kept a steady and loving presence and contributed her considerable editing skills during our co-authoring of the book.

Over the years, I have had many supervisors to whom I owe much for their gracious challenges and loving presence during varied professional roles and life transitions. I feel very thankful to Phyllis Baird, the therapist who held me through a major relationship loss and enabled me to believe in myself again. More recently, in the field of coaching supervision, I am so grateful to have been accompanied by Dorothy Allen, Margaret Lloyd and, more recently, Henry Campion and Adina Tarry.

While my involvement in establishing, supervising, and teaching on the Coaching Supervision Academy course was brief, I remain grateful to Edna Murdoch for inviting me to share in the co-creation of a programme that has developed a strong global presence. It offered me a gateway into the international field of coaching supervision.

To my clients and colleagues in the United Kingdom, Europe, Asia, and North America, mainly met through the magic of Zoom, you have all given me new ways of seeing the world and fresh ideas about the practice of coaching and supervision, for which I am enormously grateful.

The Somatic Angels – Elspeth Campbell, Louise Robb, Jackie Davis, and Terry McNerney – and I meet regularly to stretch our bodies and minds and keep alive our embodied relational consciousness, and I offer them many thanks for all we accomplish together.

My home support team has included a group of wise women: Judith Mills, Jane Inglese, Barbara Siddall, Barbara Herbin, Pat Rouse, and Barbara Wealthy. Their wisdom and love have enabled me to continue to learn from my deeper self, bringing me insights that support my continuing personal development.

My dear wife, Judith Maizels, a published author, has given hours of time and loving support, insights, and wisdom throughout the various stages of the book, particularly when at times I felt stuck and ready to give up. She helped enormously with editing throughout various stages of the book. Judith has also taught me so much about how to be in a learning and loving relationship.

Jane

First, without Fiona you would not be holding this book in your hands now. It was her vision and initiative that resulted in our beginning this conversation – initially in our respective roles as supervisor and supervisee and, as the process unfolded, as two vulnerable human beings on a mutual path of transformation. Our writing process was an exercise in passion, patience, tenacity, and determination. Throughout the entire period, Fiona offered her wisdom, loving support, and encouragement – especially during those times when I was not well enough to do any writing.

My heartfelt thanks go to Otto Vogt, my beloved partner for almost nine years. Being in an intimate relationship is a crucible for learning and development. Although we are now no longer together as a couple, our deep friendship endures.

My thoughts turn to the very able and warm-hearted psychotherapists with whom I have worked over the years, particularly Patricia Bowery and Brian Graham. Their loving holding enabled me to explore the narrative of myself mirrored in all the relationships in my life and they have contributed so much to the process of cultivating a loving relationship to myself.

I am grateful to all my coaching clients and to those mindfulness-based teachers and coaches I have had the opportunity to supervise. It is a privilege to be invited into someone's world and, through a mutual process of learning, to flex and expand the mind and open the heart. I have grown so much and continue to grow through this work of service.

Chapter 1

Introduction

Introduction

We – Fiona and Jane – wrote this book because we are passionate about our commitment to our own development as supervisors and coaches. This involves learning more tools and theories to broaden and build our professional competencies. It also includes attending to processes that support our becoming who we really are so we can offer our true selves to our clients, to work with and to relate to them.

Our primary intention in writing this book is to illustrate how, in practice, a mindfulness-based relational approach changed the quality of our supervisor–supervisee relationship and deepened our capacity to learn together. In support of this, we show that supervision relationships that are co-created challenge us to be open to generative and emergent experiences. The personal capacities and meta skills required to stay open to this way of being relational need time to develop. Learning to be relational requires that both parties are on both an inner and an outer journey of exploration.

The account of our supervision relationship is one that goes beyond what many may regard as conventional. We have developed a post-conventional supervision partnership through a range of learning contexts and role relationships, which include facilitator–participant, coach–coachee, and co-authors reflecting on our dialogical process.

I, Fiona, was inspired to write this book as a follow-up to a chapter that was published in Robin Shohet's (2011) book on transformational learning, where I referred to my work with Jane (Adamson, 2011), which was developed further (Adamson, 2012, 2013). Jane brought the skill of relational mindfulness to our

DOI: 10.4324/9781315161280-1

working relationship, opening my eyes to the potential for reciprocal learning and the developmental opportunities for supervisors themselves. In relational work, both supervisors and coaches are engaged in a process of reciprocal influence: we are learning about our capacity to stay in contact, to give and to receive, and to develop our potential for change (Cavicchia and Gilbert, 2019). Outside the therapy literature, I had not seen much acknowledgement of reciprocity, with one notable exception being De Haan, who published two collections of the results of his students' reflective inquiries into their coaching relationships (De Haan, 2012, 2016).

Revisioning

Originally, Jane's contribution was limited to the case study in Chapter 4 and our mutual reflections on our learning process. We experienced significant delays in the completion of our manuscript, largely due to Jane's periods of illness and incapacitation, about which she writes in Chapter 3. Fiona also contributed to the delays when she experienced periods of tiredness because of a heart condition and some minor health problems, which influenced her confidence in her capacity to write. As a result, we were unable to meet the deadline we agreed with the publisher and needed to repeatedly request further extensions to our submission date. Although challenging for both of us, we appreciate that our experience and understanding of dialogical relationships has deepened through our extended inquiry. This also changed what we chose to write and how we wrote, and we feel this has enriched our book. Pertinent to the time delay, we wrote our case study four years ago and this was the first part of the book to be written.

During this extended timeframe, we both came to realise that the book needed to be co-authored to render it an authentic expression of our reciprocal relational process. As a result, we made some significant changes to the structure and content of the book, deciding that all the chapters except for Chapter 6 would be co-written. In Chapter 6, Fiona writes from the depth and breadth of her experiences in the field of postgraduate education and training.

Structure

In Chapter 2, we introduce the theoretical foundations of our transformational learning process, which include Bowlby's theory of attachment and child development, Kegan's adult development framework, and relational mindfulness – the bedrock of our learning process. We include this early into the book in the hope that it will facilitate a deeper appreciation and understanding of the depiction of our relational learning process in Chapter 4 and our reflections in Chapter 5.

Chapter 3 is titled 'Coming Home to Ourselves'. Much has been written about the value of writing and sharing stories to raise self-awareness, deepen appreciation of difference and unite us in our common humanity. Aligning with this wisdom, we offer you a transparent personal account of the stories of our respective learning journeys to illustrate how we were shaped as individuals and how we contributed to each other's growth. In our individual narratives, we share what growing up has been about for each of us. We write of the many times in our lives when we have been challenged by life events, yet have been transformed by them. The process of writing evoked much grief and tenderness in each of us at times. We know that our experience is not unique, as loss and change continue to challenge all of us as we journey through life.

Chapter 4 introduces our case study, the heart of the book. Here we share our experience of how a mindfulness-based relational approach facilitates a reciprocal learning journey. Through our jointly written detailed analysis, we invite you to enter the world of a supervision relationship as it was experienced from moment to moment. We share our vulnerability, highlight our breakthroughs, and explore what enabled us to reveal that which had previously been hidden and had blocked the flow of our work. We offer vignettes of our learning journey to illustrate how we created the kind of dialogical supervision relationship that brought about transformational learning for both of us. Fiona's reflections on each of the vignettes is somewhat lengthier than Jane's. This is a remnant of the original form of our book, which we decided to leave intact to preserve the richness it offers.

In Chapter 5, we offer a meta-perspective of our learning journey. We explore attitudes, qualities and processes that facilitated a shift in our relationship, from a conventional transactional relationship to a post-conventional dialogical relationship cultivated through mutuality.

In Chapter 6, Fiona discusses the education and training of relational practitioners. She challenges what she sees as the imbalance in some current approaches to education and training, and makes the case for placing the personal development of the learner equally alongside learning of models and tools. She also explores the curriculum and assessment challenges involved and, finally, proposes the adoption of a contemplative and relational pedagogy that facilitates the development of relational practitioners.

Content of the book

While we have become particularly interested in the *how* of supervision, we are not atheoretical. The material presented here views supervision relationships through several lenses that are derived from our rich theoretical background, which informs our practice. However, ideas are also gleaned from our reflections on many years' experience in relationships of many kinds – some fulfilling and some difficult, both professionally and personally.

This book is written for you if you are a coaching practitioner, supervisor, trainer, or trainee, and for those of you in other helping relationships who wish to explore and reflect on the value of developing authenticity, often a neglected aspect of supervision relationships; discover and make sense of what helps and what hinders relational work; and consider ways to develop meta skills that will enhance and support the process of co-created learning partnerships.

We have included a few questions at the end of each chapter to offer you the opportunity to reflect on the content and relate it to your work as a relational practitioner. As you read through the chapters, we invite you to pause frequently for reflection, noticing what thoughts are arising and connecting with what you might be feeling emotionally and somatically.

References

Adamson, F. (2011). The Tapestry of My Approach to Transformational Learning in Supervision. In R. Shohet (ed.), *Supervision as Transformation, A Passion for Learning*. London: Jessica Kingsley, pp. 86–103.

Adamson, F. (2012). Looking at Coaching and Supervision Through the Lens of Love. *The Listener, A Journal for Coaches New Series, 2*, 14–18.

Adamson, F. (2013). Core Elements of Integrative, Relationship-Based Work. *AICPT, 3*, 19–25.

Cavicchia, S. and Gilbert, M. (2019). *The Theory and Practice of Relational Coaching: Complexity, Paradox and Integration*. London: Routledge.

De Haan, E. (2012). *Behind Closed Doors, Stories from the Coaching Room*. Faringdon: Libri Publishing.
De Haan, E. (2016). *Behind Closed Doors, Stories from the Coaching Room 2016*. Faringdon: Libri Publishing.
Shohet, R. ed. (2011). *Supervision as Transformation: A Passion for Learning*. London: Jessica Kingsley.

Chapter 2

Mindfulness-based adult transformational learning in theory

Introduction

The metaphor of the voyage of discovery (Proust, 1923) is apt when we think about the many challenges and changes we encounter during our journey through life, and what we may or may not learn about who we and others are becoming as we engage in supervision relationships. Will we be able to develop new eyes as we see what the world around us looks like, and can we appreciate that others may see the world differently? Are we equipped to transform who we are and how we think as we face and grow through the inevitable losses and changes of life, and are we even open to learning? Do we need to be to be on a Proustian journey to become effective relational practitioners? This chapter is our answer to this question.

Drawing on our experience of our supervision relationship, we suggest that transformational learning is influenced by two interrelated elements: our capacity to relate to others, which is determined by our early attachment styles; and our stage of adult development, which shapes the lens through which we see and make meaning of the world. With the meta skill of relational mindfulness, we believe both these elements can be transformed. A relational mindfulness approach can establish an emotional climate that is conducive to the emergence of a compassionate dialogical process, and it is this mutual process that creates the freedom to learn. It potentiates the expansion of our cognitive capacities and meaning-making frameworks, and can be a contributory factor in healing our attachment wounds.

DOI: 10.4324/9781315161280-2

Mindfulness: the foundation of relational learning

Presence or mindfulness is the cornerstone of a dialogical relationship. In its essence, mindfulness is the capacity to pay attention, intentionally, with interest, to what is happening in our present-moment experience. This includes an awareness of intrapersonal processes such as thoughts, emotions, body sensations, and impulses for action. Mindfulness also includes external sensory inputs such as sounds, sights, and the environment around us, of which a significant part is the awareness of relating to another human being.

With the practice of mindful awareness, certain qualities emerge naturally. These include being an impartial, open, non-judging witness to our experience, which enables us to be fully present and able to reflect at the same time; resting in the wisdom of patience, knowing that things will unfold in their own time; and accepting, by seeing how things are now without trying to force situations to be the way we would like them to be (Kabat-Zinn, 2013). These attitudes support a fundamental shift in our relationship to our inner phenomenological world. Rather than striving to change or avoid aspects of our experience, particularly the unwanted, we are encouraging our mind and heart to turn towards experience and meet it 'just as it is', with kindness and compassion. Through developing the capacity to pay attention to our experience in this way, we are more able to connect with how we are, without resistance.

The practice of mindfulness helps us to attune to ourselves in the moment with increasing balance, calm, insight, and acceptance. We become aware of the changing aspects of subjective experience and gain insight into our patterns of conditioning. This process encourages a shift from seeing ourselves as a static object to perceiving ourselves as part of an interdependent process intimately connected to the changing contexts of our lives.

In neurobiological terms, we are cultivating the capacity to be able to regulate our nervous systems – to dampen down the reactive flight/fight threat mechanism and activate our parasympathetic calm and connect mechanism in relation to ourselves and our inner world (Porges, 2011). This ultimately creates an inner anchor of safety. Trust in our intuition and our own authority grows from this soil.

Mindfulness is traditionally a solitary practice, and to some extent the skills we cultivate can be transferred to and exercised directly in our real-time human interactions. However, the reality is that we are highly sensitive social creatures, and connecting with our fellow human beings is inherently challenging. When our unique conditioned wounding sparks another's conditioned wounding, we are both triggered out of the present moment and into a past-conditioned dance of emotional and behavioural defensiveness. It is here that our personal relational histories, traumas and attachment styles are enacted in the present moment. When we are awash with powerful emotions and compelling thoughts, we lose sight of the person we are with, as they take on the face of our filters, projections, and assumptions. This unconscious flight/fight reactivity serves to reinforce our relational conditioning, perpetuating painful relational patterns.

To be able to stay present, to be aware that we have been relationally triggered and then to respond appropriately to the actual present moment reality can be a significant challenge! Born from our individual and mutual experience, it is our conviction that the application of mindfulness relationally can support this challenge directly.

The beauty and power of this practice lie in practitioners being supported to mindfully connect to aspects of their subjective experience that are related directly to being in a relationship – the relationship itself triggers the emergence of conditioned relational patterns. Each person supports the other's capacity to stay present, connected to the body and steady in the arising of this relational material. Through seeing these patterns emerge clearly with the clarity of mindful awareness, we are less caught up in them, less identified with them. Wisdom and compassion naturally arise from this clarity.

Relational mindfulness practice also offers the possibility of dropping below these conditioned relational patterns into a transpersonal place of heart-opening meeting. Kramer (2007) refers to the nature of this relational phenomenon as a moment of unconstructed intimacy, where our egoic defences let go and deep relational contact is possible. Martin Buber (1937) called this the 'I–Thou' meeting. Here there is regard for the person exactly as they are, in the present moment. This is a moment of radical acceptance – the elixir of true mutuality. Both can be as they are, together. In moments like this, we are one. This is the point of contact beyond individual identities, the 'between'. Hycner (1991: 30) refers to this as 'breaking out of self-encapsulation into the nakedness of direct human inter-subjective encounter'.

Early relational learning and attachment styles

All human beings have a biological need for attachment throughout life. How we think and make sense of the world was initially influenced by the kinds of relationship we had with those who cared for us at the beginning of our life. During our pre-verbal learning phase of development as infants, we experienced the emotional climate in our family as basically safe or unsafe (Erikson, 1963). When our early primary relationships have met our relational needs, we feel safe enough in the world and develop the capacity to be intimate and trusting. These are the conditions that are necessary for the infant to develop a secure attachment style that influences their capacity to learn and develop optimally.

There will be few of us who have had an entirely secure attachment as children. When such basic needs have not been met, repeatedly or inconsistently, the infant will develop defensive strategies to protect themselves against further threats to their very survival. Conditions such as mild neglect to abuse and abandonment can profoundly affect what the infant learns about the world and how they learn. The attachment styles that emerge under these conditions include anxious-ambivalent, avoidant, and disorganised (Bowlby, 1969).

Few early attachment relationships are free of threats, small or large, short-lived or enduring. What matters for the growing child is discovering that in a 'good enough' relationship, any misattunements or ruptures with their caregiver can be repaired (Bowlby, 1969). When the disconnections are not repaired effectively, most of us will grow up with unresolved emotions, fear, and insecurities about ourselves and those with whom we are in a relationship.

The learning we do in our very early childhood is largely outside our conscious awareness. We become socialised into what it means to be a member of this family, at this time in the history of our society and culture. We learn what is expected of us and how we should behave to stay safe and protected at this very early stage of our development. Our brains carry this early learning in our implicit or procedural memory, stored in a bank of data that will continue to drive our behaviour into adulthood (Trevarthan,

1993; Tronick, 2007). This memory bank informs what our essentially implicit assumptions, expectations, beliefs, and values are about ourselves and others. Such assumptive worlds, which Fonagy (2012) terms our 'mental models', may remain intact in our implicit memory until we are challenged by the inevitable losses, changes, and difficulties that life brings, and we feel a need to review them.

Because early social conditioning has inevitably involved shaping ourselves to fit in and be accepted, as adults we may hold some naturally arising but unexpressed emotional energy in our bodies. For instance, in some families the expression of feelings – either loving or angry – is not allowed. The emotional climate in some families may be icy, fiery, or even deadening to members. Such climates may trigger a shock or freeze response. Experiences such as these are felt in the body as flows of energy, and are not registered consciously by the mind, so they are very rarely spoken of (Schore, 2001). The body then carries this fear and anxiety. As a result, our attachment memories of distress and trauma are stored in the right brain as it is being developed during the first three years of life. Until our left brain is developed, sometime between 18 months and two years, we do not have the capacity to regulate our emotions. (Maizels and Adamson, 2015; Siegel, 2012). This is the period where the baby is completely dependent on the mother for regulating their nervous system, via a process of emotional co-regulation. For many of us, the impact of such flows of energy triggered early in life will have influenced our body's capacity to stay steady. For example, we may find ourselves feeling uneasy in a new learning situation and unable to manage our anxiety sufficiently to stay present. When we cannot keep ourselves in a dynamic state of homeostatic balance, of coherence, with all systems in the body operating in concert, our ability to regulate our emotions is affected and this will impair our capacity for learning. Our neurobiological systems remain in a non-integrated state (Siegel, 2012).

Allan Schore (2001), commenting on the early stages of brain development, states that

> well before the left hemisphere matures, the critical non-conscious processing functions of the right brain are well established and indeed, central to the child's adaptive affect regulation, cognition and memorial capacities. Non-conscious internal working models of attachment stored in the right brain are used by the developing psyche to dynamically interact, on

> a moment-to moment basis, with the internal world of other humans.
>
> (Schore, 2001: 270)

When the right brain is focused on surviving by mastering the current situation, we cannot switch across to access the left brain until the threat is no longer perceived. Only when we feel safe in a relationship can our brain stop triggering the cascade of stress hormones into our body, allowing us to be in a settled state, present with what is in the moment. Only then can we shift from being reactive to being responsive, and by linking the two halves of the brain we gain access to the prefrontal cortex and to our cognitive capacities.

In summary, our early learning experiences are relational. We learn first about who we are and how to be in the world through being in relationships with our parents and family, and this shapes our relational neural networks. Our minds, both inside our bodies and in the world, are then thus embodied and embedded in the social matrix. It is through these unconsciously embodied and socially embedded ways of interaction that we develop our internal working models or frames of reference. These guide our view of ourselves and how we believe we need to be in the world as we grow into adulthood. Because these processes are unconscious, it means we are unlikely to be aware of these sources of influence on us. It is our challenge as adults to come to know these sources, to learn about them and to use this new awareness to help us to make choices about how we are being in relationship.

The liminal space: a place of possibility in adult learning

From his close observations of mothers and infants, Winnicott (1988) saw that pre-verbal learning took place in the space between them, a transitional space or a liminal place of possibility, where co-created play was the medium. Play in such a space has experimentation and reciprocal learning within it, and can form the basis of a template for future learning where safety and security are present.

Being in a learning or work relationship involves giving and receiving feedback in a way that may not always be relational (Lewis, 2020). For optimal learning to occur, we need heartfelt psychological safety within an attuned and secure-base relationship (Fleming, 2008). The capacity to provide a secure base for learning requires a supervisor with the capacity to facilitate psychological safety. Without an emotional climate of safety, the potential for shame is likely to be present and may be triggered. When the insecurely attached child learns that their behaviour is seen as bad or wrong, shame emerges and is unconsciously held in their implicit right brain memory. In a supervision session, the vulnerable inner child of both the supervisor and supervisee may be reawakened when they face the experience of feeling that they should be more skilled, know more, get it right or be more articulate than they are. When this happens, a supervisor may become reactive and feel responsible for teaching their supervisee so they will learn what they do not know. Perhaps driven by their own discomfort, the supervisor may take on the role of expert, and in doing so miss the opportunity to pause, notice the unpleasant feelings and body sensations, and use this information in service of deepening the learning. This intuiting process, a tapping into the intersubjective field, is facilitated by a relational mindfulness way of being. And, through choosing to share their sense of discomfort, this can potentially open a dialogical process where both the supervisee and supervisor can explore what is being experienced in 'the between', in the here and now.

At such times, and within the container of an emotionally safe relationship, the supervisor can support themselves and the supervisee to move towards acceptance of the reality of the vulnerability of their shared human condition through mindful presence. A supervisor might say it is often like this when we learn, and it is like this for me too: there is no wrong or right way of doing things – this is what can happen when our childhood attachment wounds are triggered in a learning context; it's understandable, it's not our fault and it's okay. When we can meet mindfully, relationally, repeatedly in this learning-intensive framework, we may begin to develop a new kind of relationship with ourselves and each other. A compassionate acceptance of who we really *are* as opposed to who we believe we *should* be can emerge and we are able to become more trusting of our own judgement, our own views, our intuitive sense.

With the awareness that relational mindfulness offers, we each can learn to find our own true shape. This is where the alchemy lies. We are in the process of both transformational learning and development, moving towards potentially developing a secure attachment relationship to ourselves and finding the self-agency associated with a post-conventional way of being.

Adult development: a new consciousness emerges

We believe that, in adult life, learning to become compassionate and loving towards oneself involves releasing ourselves from our unconsciously embedded mental models – our inherited assumptions, beliefs and values about ourselves and others. This process evolves our consciousness, and we can hold a more expansive and nuanced view of the world and of ourselves. This influences how we make meaning of and respond to the life events within us and around us.

In their work on adult development, Kegan and Lahey (2009) describe moving from conventional to post-conventional levels of making sense of the world. They describe three kinds of change in adult cognitive and emotional development, beginning with the socialised mind, then the self-authoring mind, and finally the self-transforming mind.

The socialised mind is a level of consciousness where we unconsciously imbibe and live by the ideas, perspectives, and values defined by groups such as our profession, culture, and religion. We judge ourselves against the inherent standards and procedures of these social structures, striving to do things the right way. We also tend to focus on how we think others will perceive us and orient our behaviour towards that which is socially accepted and rewarded. The socialised mind is shaped originally during childhood, and the process continues into adulthood. Kegan suggests that around 60–65 per cent of the adult population do not move beyond this developmental stage.

If our life circumstances offer us conditions conducive to ongoing growth and development, we may cross the threshold into a post-conventional frame of reference. In the territory of the self-authoring mind, we create our own internal system of values and beliefs, which guide and shape our lives. Here we are able to step back, generate our own views, evaluate and make choices, self-direct, and be open to learning and development.

A small percentage of adults evolve to the self-transforming mind stage of adult development. Here, people discover that they are inextricably connected to the contexts or surrounds of their lives – there is a reciprocal relationship between these contexts and the evolving self. This is the natural playground of complexity. Characteristics of this stage include the capacity for pluralistic thinking, the ability to rest in the tension of paradox, shifts in self–other concepts towards compassionate acceptance, openness to dialectical thinking and the capacity to stay with uncertainty, ambiguity and not knowing. It also includes sensitivity to context and the ability to evaluate one's own values and views. Life becomes a learning experience and growth, and change is constant (Berger, 2018).

The evolution of consciousness may lead to a level of being that transcends the boundary of individuality and separateness. The non-dual teacher Adyashanti (2008: 69) describes it in this way:

> Until the whole world is free to agree with you or disagree with you, until you have given the freedom to everyone to like you or not like you, to love you or hate you, to see things as you see them or see things differently – until you have given the whole world its freedom you'll never have your freedom.

Mindfulness can be considered a methodology that creates the necessary conditions for vertical development through building the capacity to objectively perceive aspects of our subjective experience (Petrie, 2013). In essence, this is *relating to* experience in a subject-object sense rather than *relating from* experience where we are lost in the subjective position, entangled in the experience, with no capacity for perspective, self-reflection, and learning. According to Kegan and Lahey (2009), this is the essential mechanism in the evolution of the self to higher states of consciousness and awareness. Intrapersonal mindfulness fosters the ability 'to see, to hold ourselves closely just as we are' (Santorelli, 1999: 20). Relational mindfulness also enables us to notice and feel into our subjective experience within the mutual safety of a dialogical relationship. Significantly, we can see and hold ourselves as relational beings, just as we are.

Shifting frames of reference

During education and training, we are in a process of building our knowledge and skills – our horizontal development. One of the challenges for all of us as adult learners is to become aware of the kinds of ways we have learned to adapt to the demands of early childhood and how our minds may be shaped by our socialisation.

With a socialised mind, we are caught up in looking for others to validate who we are. To attend to our vertical development, we need to be able to notice *how we are being* in the world, step back from the received wisdom of our trainers and educators, and begin to generate our own ideas. As we develop, we may move into a transitional phase where our conventional word views begin to change. This is an inherently disruptive and destabilising period of growth, where old frames of reference begin to shift and change. Moving into the territory of the self-authoring stage of development frees us from needing others to validate who we are. We validate ourselves instead.

Our frame of reference or developmental stage will affect how we relate and how we learn. For example, the socialised mind could describe the supervisee, who is fresh out of training and at the stage of embedding the learning, concerned to do the right thing and gain confidence in using their tools and models. At this stage, supervision is about relationship building with a focus on facilitating the supervisee's capacity to apply the learning that comes from reflecting on their practice and managing their anxieties about being beginners. Starting out on a career as a coach or a supervisor in training may well be both an exciting and an anxious time because we are being asked to think not only about what we are doing but why, to become curious about our assumptions. This is the positively disruptive process of learning.

In the socialised mindset, we all carry some immunity to change where we are held back by our fears and beliefs associated with the responses of others and what they might think of us (Kegan and Lahey, 2009). It may be disturbing for us to expose what is holding us back from what a part of us may wish to say or do. For example, as supervisees or supervisors, we may refrain from asking challenging questions for fear of losing the relationship by believing we could be hurting the other's feelings.

Essentially, both parties are in a liminal place, a place of possibility, as they go through cycles of change, reflecting on new narratives and perhaps, for the first time, re-evaluating the stories they have held about themselves. The supervision relationship itself becomes the crucible for learning, and relational mindfulness co-creates this place. Herein also lies the potential for both supervisor and supervisee to expand their thinking beyond the confines of the received wisdom of the coaching profession.

Transformational learning

Transformational learning is the process of expanding our cognitive capacities and meaning-making frameworks towards a post-conventional self-authoring and self-transforming mind (Kegan and Lahey, 2009).

In so many ways, the practice of supervision is about discovering new worlds, worlds not yet dreamt of by us or those with whom we relate. This process is what makes the unsettling nature of transformational learning radical, and it can understandably generate anxiety and discomfort (Aram, 2001). We can each learn and experience ourselves in new ways, and in how we are making sense of the world. We may begin to experience our way of being as more fluid and contingent, where there is capacity to stay open and curious about the world – we step out from the familiar and risk changing our worldview. Facets of our former self disappear and new aspects appear. We are in the process of changing our sense of who we are, our personal and professional self-concept, meeting our core self, coming home to ourselves. We have changed the ego–self axis (Edinger, 1992) in such a way that we have what Bachkirova (2011) calls 'ego with a soul', a time in life when we are beginning to become engaged in our spiritual development.

According to Mezirow (1991), the process of transforming our frame of reference commences with a disorienting dilemma and concludes with a reintegration into the internal working model with a new set of assumptions. Fleming (2003: 4), using an anthropological metaphor, considers our movement through change as a

> rite of passage of three stages, comprising *separation* from previous definitions dominated by perceptions of history, situation and identity, *liminal* or transitional where the confusion brought about by the first stage is replaced by the emergence of new possibilities for change and *reincorporation* where the person's rediscoveries and new knowledge are authenticated and reinforced by being communicated to significant others and by hearing their response.

Our own model of transformational learning takes a wider view by incorporating additional data from emotional and somatic experience, the conscious and the unconscious. These are all key sources of information that facilitate learning and are brought to life within a relational mindfulness-based safe and secure relationship. Relational mindfulness is the key meta skill that enables the mutual process of being grounded, present in body, mind, and heart. This facilitates the ability to attend compassionately to what is going on within the emerging conversation, however that may be.

Reflection and reflexivity

The process of learning to reflect on an event can be enhanced using Gendlin's (2003) way of accessing embodied cognition that has some similarities to the U Process devised by Otto Scharmer (2016). The U Process represents a path by which we can let go of our conscious awareness of a situation by 'dropping down' from the top of the left-hand tip of the U to the base of the U, where we just attend and wait to see what is held just below our conscious awareness. Being in this place allows new insights to emerge, enabling us to discover new ways of seeing the situation with which we began. We can then bring our new perspective back up to the surface via the right-hand arm of the U, where we can test this out. At the heart of this way of knowing is a way of being that is contemplative, not grasping after answers but rather trusting that our body holds knowledge that simply cannot be known cognitively. We then become able to engage in what Shoshi Asheri calls 'felt participation', which is movingly described in her video discussion with Roz Carroll on humanising the therapeutic relationship (Asheri and Carroll, 2015). The value of relational mindfulness practice in this regard is discussed below.

Learning new ways of thinking and being also depends on our capacity to be reflexive. What is meant by reflexivity? It is a process that involves becoming self-aware, noticing how we are thinking and feeling somatically about something that is happening in this moment, within this relationship. It includes considering what may be happening at an unconscious level in the relational field. An example of a common dynamic seems to be a mirror or parallel to that of the supervisee's relationship with their client, and often beyond that relationship to the client's wider system. Awareness of an unconscious process may be sensed somatically, or by a spontaneous image, and when we have a sense that our relational field is carrying an energy that brings new data for reflection. The meta skill of relational mindfulness creates space and time for developing the capacity for reflexivity, for noticing what is happening in the moment without judgement. This is crucial in times of relational difficulty.

When we are uncomfortable during a supervision session, this may be a symptom that we have been triggered into relational reactivity – something that can happen at any time. Triggers are threat-based, unconsciously derived emotional responses that are wired into our brains throughout our life, and that emerge without warning in the present. Such moments of noticing may launch us into a crisis of truth when we discover that we are still guided by some of our childhood stories about how we should be (Cunliffe, 2004). These events occur in all relationships, regardless of context. In such moments, when we are flooded by stress hormones and emotionally engaged in a fear/shame response, we have little or no access to our pre-frontal cortex for a rational and considered response. Perceiving a threat to wellbeing, our right brain immediately cuts us off from access to our left brain. We may have been triggered into shame about our competency or anxiety about getting it wrong. Or perhaps we may unconsciously be projecting something onto the other and reacting to this. Under these conditions, we may well lose touch with our true sense of what we are experiencing and be unable to speak of it. Within a dialogical relationship founded on trust and compassion, we may become adept at noticing when we are triggered and more able to share this experience. Shame can heal as we develop a greater capacity to compassionately reflect on our triggers together and move into a loving acceptance of our humanity.

Cultivating relational presence

A coach or a supervisor will need to take time to explore what their client brings to their time together, to listen with their compassionate heart and to create a safe relational space in which deeper exploration becomes possible. Feeling safe to explore and to learn relationally can be generated in several ways:

- When preparing to enter each supervision relationship, at whatever stage of its development, we need to bring our whole self, body, mind and heart, with our intention being to attune to self and other in a relationally mindful way. We also need bring our intention to co-create a safe space for an emergent dialogue.

- Being relationally mindful is the fundamental meta skill. It means having some capacity to be grounded and connected to the body; focused; holding the intention to allow and accept, as best we can, whatever arises in the relational field; and leaning into the inherent uncertainty of having no conscious agenda or desire to control the process. In this way of being, we co-create psychological safety and feel safe enough to explore whatever arises in the field. Without such a relationally mindful way of being it is likely that neither will be fully available to the other. This is likely to inhibit access to our integrated brain, our field consciousness, which is needed for learning, reflection, and development within the relationship.
- Derived from Insight Dialogue (ID) (Kramer, 2007), the practice of relational mindfulness is a way of being that develops the capacity for emergent dialogue. We see becoming relationally mindful as supporting a developmental process. The meta skills of ID can be mapped onto the skills of transitioning from socialised mind to a self-authored mind state: self-awareness, somatic awareness, the ability to accept oneself with compassion, openness to an awareness of the field, interplay in the relationship, listening deeply to oneself internally and externally, and speaking one's truth without fear.
- Field consciousness is developed as we practise noticing what is going on between us in the process of supervision. For example, as I (Fiona) have become more field conscious myself, I will share and comment on my bodily response to my supervisee and the story of their work. I might say that I feel tearful, or that my chest feels tight. I offer this to encourage my supervisee to take a moment to sense into their own awareness. Our experience over time begins to make field consciousness a regular part of our dialogue.
- As we become present and attuned to the body, we are open to hearing its messages (van der Kolk, 2015). When we begin to listen to the body's wisdom, to the kind of knowing that bypasses the analytical mind, we free ourselves to go more deeply into the creative and imaginative parts of our embodied mind; the body holds information implicitly and is accessed via the right brain. For example, coach supervisors can support coaches to explore and reflect on work that evokes anxiety in them, and importantly discover how much of this anxiety is being held in the coach's body for their clients. Holding

clients' unexpressed emotions for them represents a valuable counter-transference response, a parallel process, being held until their clients are ready to acknowledge and experience it for themselves. Attending somatically will be an opportunity for coaches, their clients, their supervisors, and educators to learn and practise a vital meta skill that enables us all to read the embodied brain and to come to know ourselves and others more deeply.

- 'Window of tolerance' is a term coined by Dr Dan Seigel (2012), which is now commonly used to understand and describe normal brain and body reactions, especially following adversity. The concept suggests that we have an optimal arousal level when we are within our window of tolerance. We have capacity to be with the thoughts, emotions and body sensations that are evoked in relation to events. In a relational context, when we are emotionally triggered – a naturally occurring event in relationships – either or both supervisor and supervisee may fall into a temporary reactive state of disconnection. At such moments, the work has become too big for our autonomic nervous systems to cope and we fall outside our window of tolerance. We have temporarily lost the capacity to regulate, and we move out of the present moment and out of the relationship. With relational mindfulness, we are more able to notice that this has happened and can enter a process to reconnect together. Repair involves being aware of the misattunements or ruptures, accepting that in this moment it is so, and developing the capacity to speak about it. This involves drawing on and developing our capacity to self and co-regulate. By doing so we both widen our Windows of Tolerance through improving the integration between our left and right brain (Siegel, 2010). A significant part of healing our early attachment experiences is developing our capacity to repair and learning to trust that this is possible.

The interpersonal neurobiology of learning

A neurologically integrated brain that is functioning well is flexible, adaptive, coherent, energised, and stable (Siegel, 2012). Linkages between the left and right brain that are necessary for optimal functioning cannot be made when we feel unsafe. Siegel's definition of the mind 'as embodied and relational' is important here. He describes the process of paying mindful attention to ourselves and others in ways that develop resonant relationships as mindsight. The meta skill of mindsight can promote empathic and compassionate relationships that develop integrative brain functions. Such relationships do not just affect our general wellbeing; they also generate new neural pathways that increase our cognitive ability and the capacity to regulate our emotions.

Mindsight strengthens our ability to look at our inner world, to notice what goes on and to modify how we respond to the here and now of experience. The capacity to work mindfully and relationally helps to build an integrated brain and is a lifetime's work. Acknowledging our relational autonomic nervous systems, De Losa (2011) describes this capacity of the relational mind as the outcome of what has been termed the 'neurobiology of we'. The capacity to be in touch with and to draw from our own embodied and relational wisdom reflects the stage of adult development we are in at any time in our lives, as well as our attachment styles.

Embodied cognition: becoming somatically aware

Interpersonal neurobiologists conceptualise the mind as embodied, relational, and grounded in the body (Cozolino, 2013; Damasio, 2000; Siegel, 2012). Knowledge held in the body is accessed through paying attention to what our body is sensing in the moment, allowing the implicit to become explicit.

Relational mindfulness is a key meta skill that enables us to become aware of the relational field, to sense what is happening in the moment. Another of the many ways of accessing the body's wisdom is through focusing, a method developed by the psychotherapist Eugene Gendlin (2003). In this method, we focus on a felt sense in the body that may be expressed by a physical sensation in a part of the body, and any associated image or metaphor that arises spontaneously from our unconscious mind. We can then explore each of these 'messages' from the body. By adding focusing to relational mindfulness, we enable access to field consciousness – knowledge that deepens our capacity to bring our whole selves into the dialogue.

Conclusion

Adult learning involves body, mind, and spirit as we navigate our way through the many opportunities we have to reveal and realise our true potential. The meta skill of relational mindfulness creates a secure and safe base for learning that facilitates adult development in a climate of non-judgemental acceptance of what is, and compassion for our fallible and vulnerable humanity. Within such relationships, adult learners are engaging in a process that supports the development of relational maturity, a move towards a more securely attached way of being and a greater capacity for continuous learning and meaning-making. A spiritual dimension to adult development may be enhanced when we attend to states of consciousness that herald the stage when *being* becomes more important than *knowing* and we recognise that we are part of something that is greater than ourselves.

A relationship that truly attunes and resonates for both parties is transformational because it allows us to meet one another at a transpersonal level. It is healing us to become free from the constraints evoked in us by fear and the constraints that block our misattunements, creativity and capacity to learn.

Summary

In this chapter, we explored transformational learning and suggested that relational mindfulness plays a significant part in facilitating change in supervision relationships. We explored two interlinking factors that influenced our capacity to learn – our stage of adult development and our attachment style. It is inevitable that both parties will become emotionally triggered at some point. We showed that, through the lens of mindful awareness, we are supported to stay present in such moments and can learn together to meet these tender moments with compassion for our common humanity. We suggested that this was a key factor in our mutual vertical development. We discussed brain and body consciousness, the neurobiology of learning, and the value of developing embodied awareness. With conviction, we concluded that an attuned and resonant relationship holds the possibility to heal that which has inhibited our creativity and capacity to learn.

Questions for reflection

1 Are you familiar with your own attachment style? If yes, how does this influence your capacity to be relationally present with your supervisees or your clients?

2 In your work with your supervisees/clients, what relational practices or processes are you applying or might you apply to create psychological safety?
3 What happens when you are triggered during a session with your supervisee/client? Perhaps when you feel uncertain or uncomfortable, when you think you ought to know something or be more skilled? How do you respond to this in the moment? Would you consider disclosing this in a way that feels appropriate?
4 What do you consider your learning edge in your relational work? How might you lean into this in service of your vertical development?
5 What might the circumstances be that would alert you to step back from a relationally mindful approach with a supervisee?

References

Adyashanti (2008). *The End of Your World.* Boulder, CO: Sounds True.

Aram, E. (2001). The Experience of Complexity: Learning as the Potential Transformation of Identity. PhD thesis, University of Hertfordshire.

Asheri, S. and Carroll, R. (2015). *Humanising the Therapeutic Relationship: The Transforming Power and Risk of 'Felt Participation'.* Video lecture from CONFER online module on Advances in Relational Psychotherapy.

Bachkirova, T. (2011). *Developmental Coaching: Working with the Self.* Maidenhead: Open University Press.

Berger, J. G. (2018). *Adult Development Map.* YouTube. www.youtube.com/watch?v=pQpybfAzmM4 (accessed 12 July 2020).

Bowlby, J. (1969). *Attachment: Attachment and Loss.* New York: Basic Books.

Buber, M. (1937 [1923]). *I and Thou.* Trans. R. Gregor Smith. Edinburgh: T. & T. Clark.

Cozolino, L. (2013). *The Social Neuroscience of Education, Optimizing Attachment and Learning in the Classroom.* New York: W. W. Norton.

Cunliffe, A. L. (2004). On Becoming a Critically Reflexive Practitioner. *Journal of Management Education, 28*(4), 407–26.

Damasio, A. (2000). *The Feeling of What Happens: Body, Emotion and the Making of Consciousness.* London: Vintage Books.

De Losa, P. (2011). The Neurobiology of 'We'. *Parabola,* Summer, 68–75.

Edinger, E. (1992). *Ego and Archetype: Individuation and the Religious Function of the Psyche.* Boston: Shambhala.

Erikson, E. (1963). *Childhood and Society.* New York: W. W. Norton.

Fleming, T. (2003). Narrative Means to Transformative Ends: Towards a Narrative Language for Transformation. In C. A. Weissner, S. R.

Meyer, N. L. Pthal, and P. G. Neaman (eds), *Transformative Learning in Action: Building Bridges Across Contexts and Disciplines*. New York: Teachers College, Columbia University, pp. 179–84.

Fleming, T. (2008). A Secure Base for Adult Learning: Attachment Theory and Adult Education. *Adult Learner: The Irish Journal of Adult and Community Education*, *25*, 33–53.

Fonagy, P. and Allison, E. (2012). What is Mentalization? The Concept and Its Foundations in Developmental Research and Cognitive Neuroscience. In N. Midgley and I. Vrouve (eds), *Minding the Child: Keeping Children in Mind; Mentalization-based Interventions with Children, Young People and Their Families*. London: Routledge, pp. 11–34.

Gendlin, E. T. (2003). *Focusing: How to Gain Direct Access to Your Body's Knowledge*. London: Rider.

Hycner, R. (1991). *Between Person and Person: Toward a Dialogical Psychotherapy*. Santa Barbara, CA: Gestalt Journal Press.

Kabat-Zinn, J. (2013). *Mindfulness: Diverse Perspectives on its Meaning, Origins and Applications*. London: Routledge.

Kegan, R. and Lahey, L. (2009). *Immunity to Change: How to Overcome It and Unlock the Potential in Yourself and Your Organization (Leadership for the Common Good*. San Francisco: Jossey-Bass.

Kramer, G. (2007). *Insight Dialogue, The Interpersonal Path to Freedom*. Boston: Shambhala.

Lewis, L. (2020). *Relational Feedback: Why Feedback Fails and How to Make It Meaningful*. London: Routledge.

Maizels, J. and Adamson, F. (2015). *Breakthrough for Chronic Fatigue Syndrome, M.E. & Fibromyalgia*, Vol. 1. Bushey: Wellwise Press.

Mezirow, J. (1991). *Transformative Dimensions of Adult Learning*. New York: John Wiley & Sons.

Petrie, N. (2013). *Vertical Leadership Development, Part 1. Developing leaders for a complex world*. Centre for Creative Leadership. https://mdvconsulting.co/wp-content/uploads/CCL-VerticalLeadersPart1.pdf (accessed 10 February 2021).

Porges, S. (2011). *The Polyvagal Theory: Neurophysiological Foundations of Emotions, Attachment, Communication, and Self-Regulation*. New York: W. W. Norton.

Proust, M. (1923). *La Prisonniere: 5th volume of Remembrance of Things Past*. Paris: Grasset. www.globalgreyebooks.com/captive-ebook.html (accessed 12 December 2020).

Santorelli, S. (1999). *Heal Thyself: Lessons on Mindfulness in Medicine*. New York: Crown.

Scharmer, C. O. (2016) [2007]). *Theory U: Leading from the Emerging Future* (2nd ed.). San Francisco: Berrett-Koehler.

Schore, A. N. (2001). The Effects of Relational Trauma on Right Brain Development, Affect Regulation, and Infant Mental Health. *Infant Mental Health Journal*, *22*, 201–69.

Siegel, D. (2010). *Mindsight: Transform Your Brain with the New Science of Kindness*. Oxford: One World.

Siegel, D. (2012). *Pocket Guide to Interpersonal Neurobiology: An Integrative Handbook of the Mind*. New York: W. W. Norton.

Trevarthen, C. (1993). The Self Born in Intersubjectivity: An Infant Communicating. In U. Neisser (ed.), *The Perceived self*. New York: Cambridge University Press, pp. 121–73.

Tronick, E. (2007). *The Neurobehavioral and Social-Emotional Development of Infants and Children*. New York: W. W. Norton.

Van der Kolk, B. (2015). *The Body Keeps the Score: Mind Brain and Body in the Transformation of Trauma*. Harmondsworth: Penguin.

Winnicott, D. W. (1988). *Playing and Reality*. Harmondsworth: Penguin.

Chapter 3

Coming home to ourselves

Introduction

A paradoxical reality exists in all relationships. We are separate as individuals *and* we are inextricably connected. In the case study presented in Chapter 4, we explore the development of our supervision relationship and the mutual impact of this on each of us. As a prelude to this, we felt it would be fitting to write about our individual journeys to highlight what each of us brought into the relationship. We share seminal periods and transformational experiences in our personal development, from childhood through to adulthood. Our narratives are woven together with the common threads derived from the theoretical underpinnings of Chapter 2.

Fiona's journey

> Walking each other home.
>
> (Dass and Bush, 2018)

As I reflect on my part of this chapter, I now see the journey of my life as a pilgrimage – in a sense that I am coming to understand that the path itself is its own destination. I have been travelling along the rocky road towards coming home to myself with some wonderful companions to accompany me as we have walked on our way together. I have learned that what I do and how I am being in life is not separate from who I am becoming in each moment.

DOI: 10.4324/9781315161280-3

The shaping of an attachment style and a socialised identity

I grew up in a troubled family and learned at an unconscious level that my survival depended on my being a good, kind, and helpful child. As is so often the case with early trauma, my unconscious survival strategy had depended upon being independent, apparently not needing help and focusing on my intellectual self at the expense of my emotional self. Not surprisingly, I developed an anxious attachment style (Bowlby, 1969) that must have meant, at least on an unconscious level, that when I was in survival mode I felt it was a safe way to be in the world. I developed a strong capacity to pick up emotional atmospheres, just checking to make sure I was safe. I now reframe this as my capacity to witness and sense the relational fields I am in. I can bring this capacity into my supervision relationships, helping me to be present and attuned to the ebbs and flows in our dialogues. I have developed a secure attachment to myself, a secure base from which to relate to others.

As regards professional socialisation, I have described elsewhere (Adamson, 2011) the impact on my development as a professional of being in a supervision relationship that I felt had no room for my own personal doubts and the emotional impact of the work I was doing at that time. In my first professional role, my helpfulness was valued and unchallenged and I covered over my vulnerability about being a novice working in a children's hospital with some physically and mentally very sick and disabled children and their families. Much of my training had prepared me with models and theories, and had paid little attention to helping me to get to know myself. I was not aware that the work I was being prepared for would affect me as a person. I had no real sense that I would be using my personal resources as well as my cognitive abilities. I continued to be in my professionally affirmed socialised mind, happily accepting the role of helper. As I reflect on elements of my socialisation, I can see the connecting thread from my early attachment experience to how that shaped what I brought into my professional training and subsequent career choices. Some elements of our relational style will hinder our work – commonly a need to fix, to take responsibility for clients' change. To bring awareness of attachment issues, some supervisors give new supervisees a questionnaire to complete about their family history so that both parties can explore the attachment experiences that will have a bearing on how the coach practises and on their learning capacity. For the supervisee, it will also bring some insight into the impact of family experiences on adult behaviour (Brown, 2017). My preference and experience are to come towards this topic as the relationship develops, and as it has become a safe place to explore what could be a tender part of the supervisee.

As we will show in our case study, once Jane and I shared our anxiety about our competence, we became increasingly free to acknowledge what we were still carrying from our attachment experiences that was affecting how we worked. In some instances, it can be a support to talk about a counselling or therapy approach when the acknowledgement of the impact of attachment styles needs more attention and time.

Coming into relationship with myself

In the late 1970s, I participated in some encounter groups run by Gestalt therapists and in a short time discovered one of the sources of my anxiety about conflicts of any kind. I confronted for the very first time that I was carrying experiences from childhood about myself that were preventing me from facing and dealing with conflict. This insight was a revelation to me, and it began a process of profound change in my relationship with myself. It was a powerful call that took me into therapy and eventually to train and practise as a Gestalt therapist before I eventually left academia to become a full-time therapist. My survival self had carried much fear, sadness, and anger. I was helped to release myself from the need to hide these feelings, not only from myself but also from others. My anxious attachment style began to shift towards a more secure way of being in relation to myself and others. So continued my gradual growing up, becoming more conscious, noticing when I was holding back from expressing myself authentically.

I have made time for myself to be in therapy at various points in my life – for instance, when facing my mother's struggles with alcohol and trying to care for her myself before she was eventually hospitalised. I have discovered that my wish to care for others is now no longer an unconscious need, but rather a desire to facilitate learning and development of myself and others. Adult learning that engages with the whole person in a safe environment can engage us in an emergent relationship with ourselves, hopefully free to resist taking on the responsibility for others' lives. The need to 'fix' clients can be an issue for us as both supervisees and supervisors, so exploring this concern with compassion and curiosity can free us to move beyond this need. My sub-personality 'helpful Harriet' has had a long career and is a reminder to me of how strong the need has been in me to 'fix'. I can never say she has gone altogether!

An important source of my learning to be in a relationship with myself at a deep level began in the late 1970s when I attended a working with dreams workshop. Since then, I have trained in dreamwork and, almost without a break, led and participated in dream groups. My dream group friends continue to help me make sense of the messages my unconscious brings. The insights are often startling, and at times bring clarity about current dilemmas, revealing what lies outside my waking awareness.

Discovering core relational qualities

My two experiences of therapy training, Gestalt and transpersonal therapy, have largely been based on experiential relational learning. Learning in a group, being observed while practising with fellow learners, felt excruciatingly painful at times. I would dread the Gestalt weekends. Some of the trainers were very challenging, and I often felt like giving up. The love and support of the group carried me through to the completion of the course. Readers who did their Gestalt training in the late 1970s will know that the very confronting style of the trainers was the norm. I did learn that therapy relationships are deeply affected by the ways a therapist meets their client and will dramatically affect the outcome. I noticed that when we eventually began to free ourselves from modelling our style of relating on the trainers and found our own way of being, we became free to be experimental and playful, and able to create the kind of safe relational climate that makes for optimum learning and change.

I also learned that to work together in a way that enables change, we need to be fully present with what is in the here and now, to stay with it and explore together without an agenda. I also learned to work with the body, to pick up on the subtle non-verbal cues that tell a story not yet fully known consciously. Relational mindfulness supports me to continue to develop the meta skills I learned in Gestalt training: being present, working in the here and now, and finding the freedom to be authentic and experimental moment by moment. I am finding it much easier at this stage in my life to stay relationally mindful of the here and now, to let go of my need to be helpful and to show that I am a highly trained professional. Jung reminds us to 'Know all the theories, master all the techniques, but as you touch a human soul be just another human soul' (quoted in Cintra and Guerra, 2018)

My transpersonal training was quite different, taking a soul perspective on personal and professional development. By learning a transpersonal or psychospiritual approach to therapy, I discovered an approach to the person that considers we all have an inner life and are spiritual beings on our particular soul's journey through all elements of our lives, our learning and development. Although initially trained with a Freudian perspective in psychiatric social work, I welcomed Jung's view that explored what he called 'the archetype of life' The relationships we make in therapy are then attending to the 'note of the soul' or our 'inner artist' (McCormick, 1996) and how this is expressed through dreams, waking images, metaphors, artwork, and through bodily symptoms. Such symptoms may be understood as symbols of some yet to be expressed longings held for safe keeping until the time is right to dive deeply into this undiscovered territory. What touched me deeply during that course was what a difference it made to how I experienced myself and how I worked. I learned to take a loving and reverential view of my own and others' humanity, of our struggles to come into a full realization of ourselves and wishing to be freed from the constraints of our fears. I also learned that therapeutic relationships involve reciprocal learning, a two-way exchange that is at times experienced as an 'I–Thou' moment and this way of being with others touched me deeply (Buber, 1937). The work was often meditative and contemplative as I learned to notice, accept, and allow what was there. The whole training experience took how I worked to a deeper level than before, to be a fellow traveller on our spiritual journey.

The relational qualities I developed during my therapy training were mindfully based, although the language and the practice of relational mindfulness were not yet in the therapy domain.

Shifting frames of reference: apprehending the constructed nature of reality

As I reflect on my undergraduate studies in politics, sociology, and philosophy, I remember discovering the very unsettling idea that reality is socially constructed (Berger and Luckman, 1967). I developed a new way of seeing that each of us constructs a view of reality that is true for us and is shaped by our life experiences and those with whom we interact. For example, it is the case that we become professionally socialised into being a particular kind of professional: we are shaped and constructed to have a view of reality, an identity, about what it means to be this kind of professional. Those of us who feel constrained by this version of the truth may wish to shed it to learn our own unique way. In supervision, we may well explore questions about views of reality – for example, the questions 'How do you see this?' and 'How do you think your client sees this?' acknowledge the constructivist nature of reality. By reflecting on situations that feel stuck in some way, we may find various conceptions of reality and open up possibilities for moving on with fresh eyes. For instance, the work on unconscious bias has revealed to many of us that we have implicit assumptions about people that affect how we regard and behave towards them.

Some years ago, I spent several evenings at a clay portrait sculpture class and was astonished to see that having spent several weeks looking at a model who sat in the middle of the group, our finished sculptures all resembled us and bore very little resemblance to the subject himself. One evening when I had constructed what I thought was a good facial likeness, the tutor just took my handiwork right off the clay by removing the face. This moment shocked me and yet was great learning! What I had not done was to take a 360 degree walk around the model, to see him in the round and then to work with the whole rather than the part. We had each constructed a portrait that was filtered through a face and head shape we knew very well: our own.

In supervision relationships, how much are we seeing of the person who is with us – the part or the whole? And how much are we constructing and filtering through our own lenses? Projection is an unconscious process of attributing feelings, qualities, or attitudes to another person that we are unaware belong to us. For example, in the early stages of my supervision relationship with Jane, I was not aware of feeling anxious. I had imagined that Jane might not think that I was competent enough to be her supervisor. When in my own supervision I had mentioned Jane's comment about feeling incompetent herself, we explored what my part in this could be. I recalled telling Jane at our first meeting all about my training and the models of supervision that I used in my own supervision. I espoused a relational approach, but my anxiety had stopped me.

Mindfulness: opening into an intimate relationship with myself

I have been a meditator for many years. In the 1970s I was attracted first to transcendental meditation, Sufi meditation and then to Buddhism, and began a regular meditation practice. The term 'mindful meditation' was not in use then. At the time, I began meditating without any conscious awareness that at some level I believed – and indeed wished – it would free me from the pain of my anxious attachment way of being. I know now that I was engaged in what is called spiritual bypassing (Welwood, 2002)

I went on a retreat in 1989 with Ram Dass, a spiritual teacher known formerly as Professor Richard Alpert. I sat with him one afternoon to seek guidance with a dilemma that had arisen for me during the retreat. I described feeling a strong pull to the contemplative life and at the same time a wish to be involved in the world. He sat quietly with me for a few moments and then simply said that I could live contemplatively in my life if I wished to and need not retreat from people. I had needed reassurance from him; I was not yet quite ready to make my own choices. I immediately felt at ease in my whole being, accepting his comments and no longer seeing that these parts of me needed to be in competition. His books, *Be Here Now* (Dass, 1971) and *How Can I Help?* (Dass, 1989) have been sources of guidance on living a contemplative life without needing to withdraw.

I was becoming aware that I had lived for many years partially withdrawn emotionally, and now I had no need to seclude myself in a permanent retreat after all. I felt a shift in my body that day, a settling into being more at home with both these parts of me. From that day on, my challenge was indeed to be here now and to experience how this feels moment by moment, wanting to learn how to stay intimately connected to my bodyscape – all my senses. During the retreat, Ram Dass had introduced us all to the practice of breathing through the pain and grief we had all felt as we had witnessed film footage of human and animal suffering. Breathing through is a practice that continues to help me to stay present, especially in moments of acute emotional pain. My meditations became a place to be and not a place to which to escape. I am gradually becoming more able to notice my experience as it is happening in the present, and to allow what is there to be there.

Meditation has enabled me to become consciously embodied, to develop proprioception, or bodily awareness. In one of his stories in *Dubliners*, James Joyce (1914) describes a character called Mr Duffy, who lived a short distance from his body. This was certainly true of me until I learned that my mind was in fact embodied and relational, and in a process of constant exchange of information and energy with my environment (Siegel, 2012).

I began to have access to my embodied cognition by becoming attuned to my body, to the deeper levels of knowing that are held in the body, the unspoken aspects of our consciousness that wait to be heard (Van Der Kolk, 2015). The practice of relational mindfulness has enabled me to sense the experience of my embodied mind as I engage in the flow of supervision dialogues. The body's making of even small movements or sensations may herald an unspoken feeling or idea. Common in my experience are some of the following: when my rate of breathing changes, my chest feels tight, my shoulders are reaching up to my ears, I get headaches, and burst into tears, and lastly when I find myself gazing out of the window, lost in a separate world. It is important not to interpret all such experiences, but rather to discover their meaning in the dialogue. At times, both of us may enter a time of quiet reverie, a liminal place of possibility, of emergence, of creating a new touch point. By accessing such moments and sensations, we are developing not only our own awareness but also sharing and becoming curious about them in our dialogues as we learn new levels of consciousness together.

For example, during a period of Jane's anxiety about a business partnership in which she was involved, I had noticed that I was getting caught up in an experience of my own and was not entirely free to help Jane find her way forward without my influence. My body sent me a familiar signal, of shallow breathing and flashbacks to my own experience and my feelings about it. Once I noticed the signals, I was able to hear Jane's concerns without my agenda getting in the way. As I am becoming more open to my own experience, I am freer to be with what is emerging in the relational field.

Relational mindfulness: opening into intimacy with others

There is no question that sitting on a meditation cushion can bring many insights, but sitting with another person brings us into a whole other realm of experience. Attending to the relational field may mean opening to the ebbs and flows of some upsetting feeling states, such as shame and fear, impasses, and connection breaks, then learning how to recover and restore what has been lost between us when we can. Being relationally mindful means bringing love and compassion into our relational field. Opening to a loving and secure space enables us to be with our struggles, to honour our common humanity. We are then enabled to become engaged in embodied intersubjectivity, to be involved in bringing our whole being into the relationship moment by moment, meeting our vulnerability, allowing the flow of information between us. This way of being is contemplative, slows us down, and enables us to notice how we are being in the here and now.

In the early 1990s, I had a breakthrough moment of deep relational connection with fellow students on the final day of the dreamwork course we were completing. As part of the final assessment, we were invited to bring some artwork to present to the group that represented our learning. I wanted to show that I felt that the course had revealed much to me about what I had learned from my dream sharing – in short, that I had stepped out from behind my mask as an intellectual. The night before, I had prepared a plaster cast of a mask and a short poem painted on to an A1 poster. When I took the mask out of its box, it fell to bits! So, with tears and then laughter, I just sat there with who I was, out from behind my mask, vulnerable and yet free in the same moment, experiencing no shame and with many loving affirmations from my classmates.

My literal unmasking moment, combined with therapy, meditation and, more recently, relational meditation practices, has helped me to acknowledge that we are all vulnerable and that we do the best we can with what life brings us. Revealing our vulnerability to others can create intimacy and deepen supervision relationships.

For example, the tears that came unbidden during a session with Jane provided another moment of revealing my acute vulnerability. An observer with a rule about non-disclosure of personal information might have been shocked and judgemental. Yet it happened, and the moment was held tenderly – it was not the moment to judge, but simply to be with what was happening. I learned that day not about keeping the rules, but rather how to be in the ebb and flow of a co-created dialogical supervision relationship that is held in the relational field with compassion.

Being relationally present with others is an emotional undertaking both professionally and personally. Because working contemplatively is challenging, we need ways to work with our fears and anxieties. In almost all the many kinds of group gatherings I have been in, I have felt different levels of anxiety, sometimes involving over-preparation the night before, losing sleep and at times forgetting what I had intended to say. On the personal level, I am blessed by being in a long-term intimate relationship at home, in which we have both learned to love and be loved. On a professional level, and notwithstanding the few occasions when I have felt high levels of anxiety and lost sleep, I am learning to be open to acknowledge my anxiety, restore my equilibrium and become ready to engage intimately with others.

Anxiety is often a supervision topic. It may be a supervisor's, coach's or their client's anxiety, and it can be felt directly in the body and in the way we are often plagued by our recurring thoughts. Bringing into being a mindful start to a supervision dialogue helps settle us both, or all those present in a group, into a reflective space. When anxiety is spoken of or experienced in the field, we may then engage with it. Often, by acknowledging it we may become free of it, as it has been accepted as part of our experience and not regarded as a problem to be solved. I may suggest that we find a window of tolerance (Siegel, 2010), to enable us to create a pause, to settle our nervous systems so that we can decide or not explore the anxiety. I may offer the question, 'Is this something you would like to explore with me just now?' Sometimes a brief exploration may be enough. Here, I am advocating that in supervision we and our coaches learn to acknowledge what is present so we can restore our connection as we work with our own lived experience, whatever this may be.

Relational mindfulness has enabled me to shift my consciousness back and forth to my inner and the outer relational world. My tree or core self holds my capacity to witness and to keep me alive to these movements. For example, at times in supervision I hear myself becoming an expert when this is not called for. At that moment, my anxiety has been triggered as I felt uncertain about how to go on. I am learning to pause, attend to my breathing, drop my shoulders, slow down, and wiggle my toes to ensure that my feet are firmly rooted, and planted on the ground. I share that I have noticed what I was doing. In this way, I am in the process of returning to be open to myself and the other person, and able to commit myself to whatever is arising in the process.

Cultivating compassion: learning to love myself

It was in the grounds of my boarding school while sitting under a laburnum tree one spring afternoon that I had a threshold moment. I suddenly saw a vision of a world full of light and love, and had a profound sense that I could be a part of what I was seeing. Was this experience what Maslow (1998) described as a peak experience? No matter what I might call it, the moment has stayed with me and perhaps sowed the seed for my belief that loving energy is universal and available here for all of us. We need love to thrive as human beings, at work and in our personal lives. I now see that in this vision there was a seed of love planted in me that lay dormant waiting for me to be ready to open myself fully to it. I took several years, loving relationships, and much therapeutic help to bring this seed to flower.

As I continue my pilgrimage, I am discovering new ways of being in the world, through becoming self- and relationally conscious, learning to love myself and others, and to feel compassion for my vulnerable self. I believe that these ways of being are foundational qualities to bring to our professional and personal lives. I am still developing them and realising that it is a lifetime's work.

I took part in a Cultivating Compassion course in 2020. Many of us on this course realised that there were some people, including ourselves, for whom we found it hard to feel compassion. The supporting practices were mindfully guided meditations. The values and philosophy underpinning the course were very much in tune with those of relational mindfulness and have strengthened my capacity to be compassionate in my professional and personal life. More importantly, I am now much more willing to accept that there are times when my compassionate self has deserted me completely. The recorded meditations are available and help at such times. I am still learning to feel compassion for my flawed self.

Our vulnerability, our fear about our lovability, has roots in our attachment experiences. Until we can explore these, and some of our deepest fears, we are not free to bring love into our professional life. When we conduct our supervision relationships with love and compassion, our fears can be explored and healed.

Robin Shohet is a compassionate workshop leader doing inspiring work to bring love into his professional relationships. He shares this view of leadership with the director of the Tavistock Institute, Eliat Aram, who spoke with her colleagues at a lunchtime talk saying that, 'Compassionate leadership would be that which works with – not against – not knowing, uncertainty, ambiguity, frailty. All these exist in love.' In his writing on love and fear in supervision training Shohet regards supervision as a spiritual practice (Shohet and Shohet, 2020).

Shifting frames of reference: stepping out of the blame paradigm into self-responsibility

In an encounter group in the 1970s, I confronted for the very first time that I was carrying stories from childhood about myself that were preventing me from facing and dealing with conflict. I had been going through a very tough stage that I believe some of us go through when we rage at our parents – about how they should have taken better care of us, and why on earth did my father sign up in wartime as a soldier and then get himself killed. I now know that whatever happens, it is my responsibility and choice about how I see and feel about what has happened and is happening. I grieve for the loss of my father and for my mother's pain at loss of her husband, which she tried to soothe with alcohol. I am now able to feel love and compassion for them both. It is just as important that I feel this for myself too. I was sharing my feelings about my father with his sister, a very loving aunt, at the time of her 90th birthday. I asked her what she thought was the most important thing she had learned in life, and she said it was to love and be loved. I have been, and continue to be, loved by many people such as my aunt who are not afraid to speak of love.

I am learning to explore with love and compassion what lies behind judgements and blaming. Shifting frames of reference is a key part of supervision. Blaming a supervisee for being judgemental about a client is a sure way to induce shame. I think that if we feel compassionate as a supervisor, we can find the right way to address judgements that fit the actual situation and not look for a rule about what to say. There will be a story behind the judgement. A recent example revealed to a supervisee that he had found the work challenging and was blaming the client.

A new consciousness emerges to becoming self-authoring

Becoming self-authoring has been gradual. My professional education in clinical social work in the 1960s socialised me into my role as an expert helper, and as seeing myself as having worth through helping. I can now see that being an expert validated my role as the helper I learned to be as a child, and kept me at arm's length from clients. I felt identified with my new role and responsibility. My sub-personality, 'Helpful Harriet', found a role for herself and legitimated a part of me in my role as an expert. I was now firmly gripped in my socialised mind.

Unable to cope with the emotional demands of my first professional social work role, I escaped into academia, responding to an invitation to apply for a lectureship in a sociology department that ran a postgraduate social work course. Oh, the irony of being 'head hunted' as if this was the only part of me being invited into academia!

Movement towards becoming self-authoring was initiated by my involvement in the development of a small new business. As the business developed, our working relationships became strained. I also felt I had failed to stand up for what I believed and valued. I now see that I escaped from the conflict among us, unable – for my part at least – to contribute to any kind of resolution. I think now that my early family script was being played out, 'Fiona the helper' in a conflict situation that she could not resolve on her own.

I had to find my own voice. This very painful event gave me the impetus to take the step I needed to shift towards becoming self-authoring. I needed to find my own future way in my chosen profession, and then to step out into the unknown. My dear supervisor at the time had given me Mary Oliver's (1986) poem 'The Journey', which really resonated with me and made me feel supported in my decision to begin walking my own path. I saw that the time had come when I needed to follow what felt right for me, as expressed so beautifully in Derek Walcott's (1976). poem 'Love After Love', ready to greet the stranger who was myself.

Shifting frames of reference: illness as a spiritual teacher

My body was a much-neglected part of me for many years, and held much unexpressed fear, anxiety, and anger that had been stored during my childhood. I had to have major surgery in my late forties and took several weeks' convalescence to recover my strength. During that time, I realised how much I had neglected some of the earlier symptoms that had suggested all was not well physically. I learned that there's a real difference in knowing you have a body and really coming into a relationship with it. I felt vulnerable as I left convalescence for home. Paradoxically, I was also relieved that I felt ready, stronger in my whole being, and that I had a body I wanted to take care of. I needed to take care of my whole being. This stage brought me closer to loving my embodied self than I had ever been before. It also reminded me that to hold all of myself in love is a spiritual practice. It means that when illness took me out of my everyday responsibilities, and I had no choice but to accept this and to hand over to others to care for me. I discovered that accepting help felt right and good – a step towards knowing that we are all interconnected and owe our lives to this fact. I moved willingly out of my self-sufficient self.

I have learned to inhabit my body as well as my mind, and to find ways to attend to life from my core. My learning to meet again the stranger who was myself has taken many years, guided by many people, experiences and relationships to bring me home to myself: a human being on a spiritual journey. I continue to be a journey companion, walking with others towards home.

Jane's journey

Here I describe my personal journey towards becoming a mature adult and a more embodied human being. I explore the evolution of the relationship with myself, and how mindful awareness and compassion have softened the conceptual narratives and beliefs characteristic of the anxious attachment and socialised mind patterning. These parts of my life's journey reveal the rocky and sometimes treacherous terrain that I've traversed to be able to find the path home to my authentic self. Even during the darkest nights, I connected with the sense of a process unfolding and was aware that there was something much greater at play than I could understand.

I have divided my writing into interrelated sections that follow a linear timeline of significant psychological and spiritual life events. I describe the people, places and practices that have supported and are continuing to support the process of my unfolding. My narrative is written in the past tense to adhere to the timeline and facilitate ease of reading.

The shaping of an attachment style and a socialised identity

The familial conditions of my infancy and early childhood shaped my growing nervous system in an anxious-attachment configuration. In Erikson's (1994) developmental terms, the first stage of psychosocial development *trust vs. mistrust*, resolved in favour of mistrust – which is the experience of so many children. This resulted in a perception that the world was not safe and impacted my capacity to feel secure in relationships. It also impaired the relationship I had with myself – I could not be open to my experience and trust myself. Mistrust also shaped my sense of worth and I was plagued with self-doubt for most of my life. I believed that I was inherently not good enough, not intelligent enough, not attractive enough, not enough. Alongside this, I believed that if I tried hard, I would one day "get it right" and be regarded as good enough. Then I would be worthy of being loved.

I began identifying with a false adapted sense of self to meet external conditions of worth – I must be intelligent, good, quiet, funny, slim, attractive, motivated, driven, ambitious; I should strive for excellence, excel academically, have a car, own a house, look a certain way, wear certain clothes ... The qualities of this self were also inextricably conditioned by my culture, Western society, education, heritage, and environment. I lived inside this sense of myself for a good part of my life, doing the best I could to fit in, to belong, be seen, acknowledged, validated, accepted, and loved.

During my transition into early adolescence, my mother provided me with the support and structures I needed to develop my musical talent. Mum identified that I had an unusual musical aptitude and the gift of perfect pitch when I was three years old. However, it wasn't until I was 13 that the circumstances of my life supported the nurturing of this talent. From then until I was in my early twenties, I practised the piano or the organ for three to four hours each day. The combination of talent and discipline was met with much success and recognition. I won many prizes at competitions and, at the age of 16, was chosen as one of eight to play with an orchestra for the Young Person's Orchestral Festival, held annually. I also learned to play the organ, took on the role of the organist for the university choir, and gave an organ recital in the city hall in Johannesburg in the final year of my Bachelor of Music degree.

This period of my life enabled me to demonstrate my talent to society and, most importantly, win approval from many. Many of my psychological needs were met through my music, albeit at quite a cost. Classical music demands perfection in its execution. I spent hours of every day working to perfect the technical and interpretive aspects of my repertoire. Developmentally, during this time a person's sense of identity or self-concept is establishing itself. The fear-based pattern of striving for perfection in an attempt to get my needs met became firmly entrenched in my false sense of self.

Coming into relationship with myself

In my late twenties, I decided to undertake the training necessary to become a voluntary telephonic counsellor for a service called LifeLine in Johannesburg. The course was structured to include 50 per cent skills training and 50 per cent personal development. The door to my inner world opened, and for the first time in my life I was confronted with psychic material that had been lying dormant, buried in my unconscious. I realised I had been living an unexamined life, and this led me into psychodynamic psychotherapy. I worked with my therapist regularly for 12 years and uncovered so much about myself. The work we did together started to erode the negative core beliefs associated with my false sense of self. We also explored the defensive relational behaviours associated with my attachment style and began to untie the knots of fear that held me captive in mistrust.

Discovering core relational qualities

Following on from the counsellor training, I had aspirations to complete a master's degree in clinical psychology at a university in Johannesburg. My personal safety felt increasingly threatened with the steady rise in crime in the country and, at the age of 37, I emigrated to the United Kingdom. I felt optimistic and excited to start a new life. My first personal development step in my new country of abode came with a foundation year in integrative psychotherapy at the Metanoia Institute in London. Here, I began to more fully appreciate and understand the potency of the therapeutic relationship. I learned about Carl Rogers' (1963) core relational conditions – unconditional positive regard, empathy, and congruence – and recognised the impact that these capacities can have on the quality of relational contact. Later, during the period of writing my master's thesis, my understanding of these conditions deepened. I wrote, 'In his later years Rogers' writing reveals the tentative proposition that the relational conditions emerge *from* the ground of presence, that being present is an embodiment of the therapeutic conditions' (Brendgen, 2014: 19). With the support of mindfulness, these core conditions shifted from concepts into lived embodied relational experience, where I was able to see the reality of Rogers' wisdom directly for myself.

I decided to pause the therapy training in favour of a coach training programme and began practising as a coach in the corporate sector. A few years later, I met Fiona and we began the journey of supporting each other's growth and development.

Shifting frames of reference: apprehending the constructed nature of reality

When I was 44, the events and circumstances of my life precipitated an existential crisis, where I questioned the meaning of everything. One of the biggest contributory factors was the despair I felt regarding the breakdown of a five-year relationship that was beset with painful attachment patterns. My sister Emily strongly encouraged me to attend a personal development programme called The Landmark Forum. This three-day course is grounded in a model of transformative learning. By way of a meticulously designed programme, participants are guided into a profound experiential process that holds the possibility for deep insight and transformation. At 3.00 pm on the last day of the course, I experienced a momentous paradigm shift. In that moment, I realised that everything was essentially empty and meaningless and that my reality and self-concept were socially constructed – made up. My whole body vibrated with rapture and I laughed with joy at this existential joke. The insight faded quite quickly; however, I experienced what felt like an altered state of consciousness for four or five months afterwards. My mind felt clear and I was extraordinarily happy. My thinking expanded beyond my existing views and limits, and I was attracted to Buddhist philosophy and mindfulness meditation. This was a remarkable time in my journey inward, towards greater self-knowing, self-acceptance, and wholeness.

Mindfulness: opening into an intimate relationship with myself

I was drawn to mindfulness, as so many are, as a way to overcome attachment relational wounding, in the hope of finding ease in my relationship with myself and to others.

Before I began practising mindfulness, I had no idea how scattered and perpetually distracted I was. When I started the practice of mindfully attending to the breath and body, I began to develop an understanding of the nature of the human mind and of why training attention is so essential. I saw that it was virtually impossible to settle, to be still and actually turn towards my experience in the moment. I understood this to be the fundamental human condition. Furthermore, relationally my anxiously attached nervous system was in a perpetual state of low-level threat. I was, for the most part, living inside my head in an abstracted world of thought.

After many years of dedicated daily practice, and many hours of retreat practice, things started to change. With the quietening of my mind, I was able to stay in the body and perceive the nature of the mind with greater clarity and less identification. Through attuning non-judgementally to the changing aspects of my subjective experience, I was developing the capacity to be more present to and for myself. By allowing my experience to be my experience, an inner sense of intimacy, safety, and trust began to develop. The beloved Buddhist teacher Pema Chodron (2020) describes the process in this way:

> We gradually drop our ideals of who we think we ought to be, or who we think we want to be, or who we think other people think we want to be or ought to be. We give it up and just look directly with compassion and humour at who we are.

Allowing or acceptance is an essential ingredient for growth, particularly in the face of difficulty. I was learning to stretch my window of tolerance through coming into an increasingly intimate relationship with whatever was here: pausing, relaxing, and feeling into the doubt, despair, anxiety, fear, jealousy, and anger; honouring what was here in the body and mind without falling into the narrative of identification and becoming it. I recognised acceptance as the necessary groundwork for developing an open authentic relationship with myself. And I regard this as the vital factor underpinning my ability to be present, connected, and trusting in relationships.

Relational mindfulness: opening into intimacy with others

The practice of relational mindfulness provided the opportunity to transfer the skills I was developing in terms of my relationship to myself directly into my relationships with others. During my first seven-day meditation retreat at Gaia House, I paused to read information pinned to the noticeboard regarding an upcoming relational mindfulness retreat. This was my first encounter with Gregory Kramer's (2007) relational practice of Insight Dialogue (ID). Intuitively, I knew that this would change my life. A year later, I attended my first ID retreat and recognised the transformative power held by this form of practice. This excerpt from an essay written for the Mindfulness and Individual Therapy module for my master's degree at Bangor University (Brendgen, 2010) speaks volumes:

> Through a powerful container process (pause, relax, open, trust emergence, listen deeply, speak the truth), we are invited into mindful dialogue where we are able to observe our relational habits as they appeared in real time. Here, with the support of each other and the mutual practice of the attitudes of acceptance, compassion, kindness, curiosity and non-identification, our hearts are gently encouraged to open to the possibility of a profound encounter with another. In this sacred place I felt my ego let go of its defensive role as it came to a place of rest, allowing the authentic Jane who embodies a quality of very human relational presence that is transparent to open-hearted being, right in the midst of the dense confines of worldly conditioning, to step forth.

After this retreat, I established both an intrapersonal and an interpersonal mindfulness practice, and they complemented and strengthened one another. I also decided to go back into psychotherapy and made a commitment to myself that I would work psycho-spiritually, attending to my psychological growth and my spiritual development concurrently. I have sustained this commitment to the current day, albeit in a different form.

Through the practice of ID, I learned what it meant to be present, anchored in my body, attuned to my internal experience *while* being attuned externally, in a relationship. This was a revelation. It profoundly influenced how I related to myself in relationship and those with whom I was in relationship.

It was here that I reconnected with my true experiential self, the one that is innately capable of being present, embodied, and open to the changing flow of subjective experience. She had been waiting patiently in the present moment for me for all my life. I felt safe, grounded in present moment lived experience, free from the confining narratives of the past and the projections of the future.

The more I was able to inhabit my experiential self in relationship, the more my sense of self-consciousness, insecurity, and self-doubt faded. It felt as if I was coming out of hiding, from behind the mask of the false self. I discovered access to a deeper wisdom through the gateway of the body and, for the first time, I found my authentic voice. I noticed my thinking and speaking moving from my head and more into my body; the pace of my speaking slowed and my voice became more resonant. A sense of my own authority and quiet confidence was born out of this place, and it was effortless. It happened organically – I didn't have to try to actively change myself. The core belief that plagued me for most of my life – that I was not good enough, and particularly that I was stupid – began to fade and lose its power. I started to connect with the reality of my strengths and human limitations, with appreciation, compassion, and kindness rather than with inflation, judgement, and shame. It became increasingly comfortable to speak openly about my human failings, with lightness and humour.

I noticed that the way I related to others was also changing. I could lean into the uncertainty inherent in each relational moment and be with what was arising, riding the dynamic flow of relating. This included being more able to stay grounded in the moments of discomfort, reactivity, and disconnection so characteristic of human relating. I noticed my heart becoming more compassionate as my window of tolerance grew. I also noticed that there was increasing ease of connection. Resting in receptive presence, I was more able to perceive others through a clear, present-focused lens rather than through an opaque, past-based narrative lens. With a past-based lens, my own history – conditioned thoughts, preconceptions, prejudices, opinions, judgements, assumptions, expectations, and beliefs – is very likely to be unconsciously projected onto the person with whom I am relating. When this happens, I am no longer seeing the person; rather, I am seeing my own reflection. Perceiving someone through a present-focused lens is radically different. In his book *Stillness Speaks* Eckhart Tolle (2003) describes this as the process of giving our fullest attention to whoever we are interacting with. Consequently, we take the past and future out of the relationship and relinquish the conceptual identity we constructed for them.

Presencing in this way sensitised and expanded my listening and perceptual capacities to include everything in the phenomenological field – my sense experiences, the whole body, emotions, thoughts, the other person, the environment, and the context within which the interaction was taking place.

Shifting frames of reference: cutting the ties of perfection

Completing a thesis for a master's degree at Bangor University taught me so much on so many different levels. I attended an ID retreat during the period when I was considering what topic to focus on. The topic of authenticity emerged while I was engaged in dialogic meditative practice. I saw this as an imperative call, to embark on the 'Hero's Journey' to find my way back to my true self. I chose to focus on the experience of authenticity in teaching mindfulness, and hoped to highlight the importance of relational mindfulness in this context. I selected heuristic research methodology, which is in essence a form of self-inquiry. The Greek root of the word 'heuristic' means to discover or find (Moustakas, 1990). It offered the potential for increased self-awareness, self-knowledge, and transformation. I quote from my thesis: 'Through daring to surrender to the (inner) listening, the constituent parts of the self are reorganized and reintegrated, and the experience of self is transformed' (Brendgen, 2010: 28).

The whole research process was an extraordinary experience, and it took me to places within myself that I had not visited. I approached this project with the discipline and focus that I had learned when I was a classical musician. The pattern of perfection and getting my needs met was powerfully activated during this time. Similarly, I spent many hours of every day striving to do my best, driven by the conscious and unconscious need to be seen and accepted. I wanted to finally prove that I was intelligent enough, good enough, worthy of being loved. The irony here was that I had chosen authenticity as my topic. I was being guided in the direction of finding my true self through the impetus of perfectionism, the antithesis of the reality of the ever-changing imperfect fallible human being that I am.

I obtained a first-class degree and was awarded the prize for being the top student in my year. The greatest rewards I received were surprisingly not these socially lauded accolades but rather the psycho-spiritual fruits of the heuristic process. A few days after the graduation ceremony, I woke up one morning and experienced a powerful embodied insight. I realised that there was no perfect accomplishment and that there could never be. There are no universally established set standards for excellence. Everything was relative, constructed, and changing. The illusion of perfection was dissolving in front of my eyes. I recognised that my socially conditioned mind had created this belief and then attributed meaning to it as if it were the truth. Joyful laughter arose from deep within my body. It felt liberating. This was another significant step in the recognition that I was in a process of waking up out of the matrix of a socially constructed reality and sense of self.

Cultivating compassion: learning to love myself

This process of getting to know and accept myself as I am has been profoundly supported by the practice of self-compassion. I attended a self-compassion retreat in October 2016, based on the work of Kristen Neff and Chris Germer (2018) and started the daily practice of intentionally being kind to myself. In combination with my psychological work, work with Fiona, and mindfulness practices, I noticed how self-compassion was helping to shift my neurobiology from threat to increasing safety, rewiring my attachment style from fear to trust. In the friendlier chemistry of safety, more of my inner parts or aspects of myself have been able to reveal themselves to the compassionate warmth of awareness. The Buddhist teacher Jack Kornfield (2000) said that maybe all spiritual life is about self-acceptance. I understand now that this is the process of bringing all the parts of myself home, moving from fragmentation to wholeness.

During this period, I encountered the compassionate work of Paul Gilbert (2010). In one of his talks, he spoke to his audience saying, 'It's not your fault and it's your responsibility.' I really got it, as an embodied truth rather than an intellectual understanding. The way my nervous system was wired when I was a child was not my fault. For the first time, I knew rather than understood that it was not personal. It was as a result of a multitude of complex causes and conditions, so many of which were intergenerational and cultural. I was finally able to see the truth of this and let go of blaming myself and others. At the same time, I saw the paradoxical truth that, although my conditioning is not my fault, what I do with it is fully my responsibility. This significant shift, supported in part by Paul Gilbert's timely wisdom, has enabled me to be much more tender and compassionate towards myself and others, particularly when I or the other gets triggered into relational reactivity.

Shifting frames of reference: stepping out of the blame paradigm into self-responsibility

A few years ago, I experienced an intensely painful and irreparable rupture with a close friend when we were both triggered into our core attachment wounds. I recognised more of my fragility, shadow, and limits, and I encountered the reality that loss is an inevitable part of transformation. The pain of this experience fuelled my engine of growth, and my perception and interpretation shifted from blame into the maturity of personal responsibility. I knew my triggers – my past playing out in the present – were not my fault, and were fully my responsibility in terms of how I responded. It became easier to recognise closer to the moment that I was triggered, to openly own it as such and to apologise for my reactive behaviour, if appropriate. Being accountable to oneself *is* sometimes an experience of intense vulnerability. When it is possible to hold our very human fallibility with compassion, paradoxically a quiet confidence arises from the ground of humility.

Similarly, I knew that most people in our world say and do what they do from their own set of socially conditioned fears, defences, and attempts to survive – and that most of it, even when aimed directly at us, has nothing to do with us and is rather more a projection of their own unresolved pain. This knowing deepened my capacity for compassion and expanded my ability to think in systemic terms and appreciate the interdependence of things. Now, when my partner, a family member, or someone I know gets triggered in relation to me, I have a greater capacity to pause and ask what is going on, to better understand what is happening for both of us in the unconscious mutual dance. I welcome relational trigger points, seeing them as opportunities to discover more about myself, possibly uncover previously unseen shadow aspects or blind spots, understand the other more fully and, most importantly, use the grist in service of deepening relational contact. I am also more adept at taking care of myself by exercising appropriate boundaries when necessary.

During this generative period, my understanding of empathy deepened based on my own experience and changing needs. I saw how it transformed in character relative to stages of adult development. It feels more appropriate to share my insights in Chapter 4, which is more theoretical.

A new consciousness emerges: becoming self-authoring

From childhood, I conformed (consciously and unconsciously) to social, community and cultural norms to be accepted, to be loved, and to feel safe. My socialised mind was trapped in the need to belong, to fit in, and I lost touch with my deepest needs and my true self. During the writing of my master's thesis, I came across a Jack Kornfield quote that became the bedrock of the work. It captures the challenge inherent in breaking free from this mindset: 'To be nobody but yourself in a world which is doing its best to make you everybody else means to fight the hardest human battle ever' (Kornfield, 2000: 213).

One of the most difficult aspects of coming home to oneself is the experience of feeling nakedly vulnerable and lonely. I appreciated the truth of this more fully when I decided to leave the mindfulness practice group of which I had been a member for many years. This was as a result of a perceived breach in the psychological safety of the group. One of the members offered me this quote to reflect on:

> The process of community building begins with a commitment – a commitment of the members not to drop out, a commitment to hang on in there through thick and thin, through the path of chaos and emptiness without that commitment community is impossible.
>
> (Peck, 1990: 300)

I interpreted this conception of community as being congruent with conventional thinking. It was predicated on the principle of subordinating one's values and needs in service of the community. At this point, I appreciated that compromising my values to be understood and accepted was more painful than being rejected. I made the courageous decision to disentangle myself from the expectations of the group, stand in my truth, and brave the wilderness of uncertainty and criticism as Brene Brown (2017) describes in her book, *Braving the Wilderness: The Quest for True Belonging and the Courage to Stand Alone*. Although very emotionally upsetting at the time, this experience was truly a gift because I realised that my choices were no longer being dictated by external conditions of worth and fear. I was finding refuge in my own values and sense of self as I walked the road less travelled towards belonging to myself.

Mary Oliver's poem 'The Journey' resonated strongly with me at this time. I intuited that she was familiar with the rocky wild territory associated with transitioning from the socialised mind into a new world. I found particular solace in recognising that there *was* a new voice emerging, a voice that I finally recognised as my own, that inner voice of wisdom and truth. This voice kept me company as I walked deeper and deeper into the world with increasing clarity and determination to 'do the only thing that I could do, to save the only life that I could save' (Oliver, 1986: 38).

Shifting frames of reference: illness as a spiritual teacher

As mentioned in Chapter 1, the writing of this book has been significantly protracted by periods of debilitating illness that started in August 2015. This began quite suddenly and without prior symptoms other than feeling very open and joyful. For a period of seven days, I was plunged into existential terror and panic and came face to face with a sense of my own mortality. It felt like I was falling apart. Before this, I had no history of mental health problems. These episodes happened once a year from then onwards, for up to two months at a time, and the most recent incapacitated me for over a year. I am still in recovery as I write these words. These experiences were likely to be caused by a host of interrelated factors, including the depletion of oestrogen in my body due to the menopause, transformational crises in the form of spiritual emergency, and a very challenging experience on a meditation retreat where there was a lack of attendance to trauma-sensitive protocols. I experienced difficulties with my daily meditation practice from that time onwards.

It was during this time that I encountered the seminal work of Willoughby Britton (Britton et al., 2017). Her research focuses on under-reported negative phenomena associated with meditation. I reached out to her and it was such a relief to be understood. I also felt somewhat consoled to learn that the experienced practitioners linked to her research were reporting cognitive, affective, perceptual, social, and particularly somatic experiences not dissimilar to mine. Of her subjects, 82 per cent reported fear, anxiety, and panic. Their associated levels of distress and functional impairment ranged from minimal and transient to severe and enduring. I am left wondering whether all her subjects experienced developmental trauma.

These periods of extreme difficulty helped me to grow and mature in ways I could not have imagined, and gave me realisations about life that can only come from the depths of suffering. I became familiar with the paradoxical truth about which many Buddhist teachers speak: preparing for death rejuvenates one's appreciation for life. I learned to find greater ease in uncertainty as I settled into the territory of 'not knowing'. During these times, I grieved for so much: my health, the work that I felt passionate about and was unable to do, and a sense that I had lost my place in the family of things. I had to completely let go of my committed formal mindfulness practice and the possibility of ever attending meditation retreats, which had been a joy for me.

I held myself with compassion every day, and experienced moments where I felt exquisitely connected to all human beings who were suffering at that very time. I felt held in the arms of common humanity, which carried me out of the depths of despair on so many occasions. I also recognised how much agency I had – that I could choose which thoughts to follow, choose in the moment what felt like the next best step to take care of myself, choose my attitude towards the difficulty, choose to stay open to experience as best I could.

These phases of illness were the darkest times of my life, yet I can see that the process of unfolding has continued. I recognise that my heart has become more tender and compassionate, a lot of my protective armour has been stripped away, I inhabit a fuller humility, and am more rooted in my true self. In the letting go of a formal daily sitting practice, my life has become my practice – washing up, cleaning my teeth, showering, chopping vegetables, listening to music, hearing the birds sing, noticing my chattering mind, recognising changing mind states, and feeling shifting emotional valences in the body, dropping into compassion during difficult moments and feeling the warmth of my hands on my heart, softening into physical pain, feeling my feet on the ground as I walk. Meeting people in the various contexts of my life offers me the richest form of daily practice. I am so deeply grateful to be able to settle into an embodied relational presence, open and receptive to what is arising here and now.

I am now on hormone replacement therapy, which has helped to replenish my physical resources, enabling me to re-engage with many aspects of my life, including this writing. I am still experiencing health challenges, and live each day with the uncertainty that I may fall into another period of illness. Today I am doing my best to be here, for now. I am deeply grateful for the miracle of life and live more in gratitude than I ever have.

Summary

In this chapter, we – Fiona and Jane – have written of our individual journeys to highlight what each of us brought into our working relationship. The themes that we used to weave our narratives together were derived from the theoretical underpinnings of Chapter 2: the shaping of our attachment styles and our socialised sense of identity; discovering core relational qualities; an exploration of mindfulness to foster intimacy with ourselves and others; cultivating compassion for ourselves; and learning to love the imperfect fallible human beings that we are. Each of us explored experiences we felt helped to shift our frames of reference and accelerated our individuation process, enabling us to disentangle from the socialised mind and find refuge in a reality that is self-authored.

Question for reflection

What were some of the seminal moments in your life that changed your perspective and how you made sense of yourself and the world?

References

Adamson, F. (2011). The Tapestry of My Approach to Transformational Learning in Supervision. In R. Shohet (ed.), *Supervision as Transformation, A Passion for Learning*. London: Jessica Kingsley, pp. 86–103.

Berger, P. L. and Luckmann, T. (1967). *The Social Construction of Reality: A Treatise in the Sociology of Knowledge*. London: Allen Lane.

Bowlby, J. (1969). *Attachment. Attachment and Loss*: Vol. Loss. New York: Basic Books.

Brendgen, J. (2010). Mindfulness and Individual Therapy. Unpublished essay, University of Bangor.

Brendgen, J. (2014). Embodied Presence: A Heuristic Inquiry into Mindfulness Teachers' Experiences of Authenticity. Unpublished master's thesis, University of Bangor.

Britton, W. B. et al. (2017). The Varieties of Contemplative Experience: A Mixed-methods Study of Meditation-Related Challenges in Western Buddhists. *PLoS ONE*, *12*(5), e0176239.

Brown, B. (2017). *Braving the Wilderness: The Quest for True Belonging and the Courage to Stand Alone*. New York: Random House.

Buber, M. (1937 [1923]). *I and Thou*. Trans. R. Gregor Smith. Edinburgh: T. & T. Clark.

Chodron, P. (2020). Six Kinds of Loneliness. *Lions Roar*, 30 July, www.lionsroar.com/six-kinds-of-loneliness (accessed 2 February 2021).

Cintra, C. and Geurra, G. (2018). *Together: The Power of Shared Business Leadership*. Lisbon: Editora Belas-Letras.

Dass, R. (1971). *Be Here Now*. London: Crown.

Dass, R. and Bush, M. (2018). *Walking Each Other Home: Conversations on Living and Dying*. Boulder, CO: Sounds True.

Dass, R. and Gorman, P. (1989). *How Can I Help?* London: Rider & Co.

Erikson, E. (1994). *Identity and the Life Cycle*. New York: W. W. Norton.

Gilbert, P. (2010). *The Compassionate Mind*. London: Constable.

Joyce, J. (1914). *Dubliners*. London: Grant Richards.

Kornfield, J. (2000). *After the Ecstasy the Laundry: How the Heart Grows Wise on the Spiritual Path*. London: Rider.

Kramer, G. (2007). *Insight Dialogue: The Interpersonal Path to Freedom*. Boston: Shambhala.

Maslow, A. H. (1998). *Maslow on Management*. Hoboken, NJ: Wiley & Sons.

McCormick, E. (1996). *Change for the Better: Life-Enhancing Self-Help Psychotherapy Approach*. London: Sage.

Moustakas, C. (1990). *Heuristic Research: Design, Methodology, and Applications*. London: Sage.

Neff, K. and Germer, C. (2018). *The Mindful Self-Compassion Workbook: A Proven Way to Accept Yourself, Build Inner Strength, and Thrive*. New York: Guilford Press.

Oliver, M. (1986). *Dream Work*. New York: Atlantic Monthly Press.

Rogers, C. R. (1963). The Concept of the Fully Functioning Person. *Psychotherapy: Theory, Research and Practice*, *1*, 17–26.

Scott Peck, M. (1990). *The Different Drum: The Creation of True Community – the First Step to World Peace*. London: Arrow Books.

Shohet, R. and Shohet, J. (2020). *In Love with Supervision: Creating Transformative Conversations*. Monmouth: PCCS Books.

Siegel, D. (2010). *Mindsight: Transform Your Brain with the New Science of Kindness*. Oxford: One World.
Siegel, D. (2012). *Pocket Guide to Interpersonal Neurobiology: An Integrative Handbook of the Mind*. New York: W. W. Norton.
Tolle, E. (2003). *Stillness Speaks*. Vancouver: Namaste.
Van der Kolk, B. (2015). *The Body Keeps the Score: Mind Brain and Body in the Transformation of Trauma*. Harmondsworth: Penguin.
Walcott, D. (1976). *Sea Grapes*. New York: Farrar Straus & Giroux.

Chapter 4

Case study

Introduction

In Chapter 2, we introduced the theoretical foundations of our transformational learning process, which included attachment theory, adult development, and relational mindfulness. In Chapter 3, we offered insight into our personal journeys, highlighting what each of us brought to our mutual learning relationship. Our narratives were woven together using common threads derived from the theoretical foundations. We hope that this information will enable you to engage more deeply with our learning journey – the heart of our book – which is expressed in this chapter.

Here we – Jane, the supervisee and Fiona, the supervisor – chart the development of our supervision relationship over the 12 years we have been working together. We explore the mutual impact of this, both professionally and personally, to illustrate how mindfulness-based relational supervision facilitates transformational learning and new ways of being. We outline the cycles of mutual change over time, including our dawning awareness of the echoes of our personal histories affecting our capacity for relational and generative learning. We write candidly about our intersubjective experiences, highlighting breakthrough moments that revealed what we had consciously and unconsciously kept hidden. We explore how our increasing willingness to reveal our vulnerability blossomed into mutual love and compassionate presence, and how this deepened our reflective capacities and shaped our learning about how we worked as a coach and as a supervisor.

We take an autoethnographic approach, using the data contained in our reflective notes and our post-hoc realisations to build a composite picture of the narrative of our relationship and our co-created

DOI: 10.4324/9781315161280-4

learning process. Adjacent to our narrative, and where appropriate, we point briefly to the theories and models that have informed how we perceived, made sense of, and plotted the developmental phases of our relationship. These references are discussed more fully in Chapter 2.

Background contextual information

Before we begin this exposition of the evolution of our dialogical supervision relationship, we offer a brief biographical sketch of each of us, to provide relevant contextual and chronological information.

Fiona

I was born a fraternal twin in 1943, growing up in a turbulent family atmosphere in post-war England.

Following a degree in sociology, politics and philosophy in 1966, I trained in clinical social work and went into the NHS to work in a multidisciplinary team in the field of child and family psychiatry in a teaching hospital. I then spent 18 years in academia to escape from an emotionally demanding role in the hospital. I loved small-group teaching, collaborated in interdisciplinary teaching and research in the medical school, and carried out qualitative research into work groups for an M.Litt. while working part-time in a general practice surgery as a community-based social worker.

I completed two therapy trainings. My first training was in Gestalt, where I learned to work experientially in the moment. I then added a psychospiritual perspective to that way of working through attending a transpersonal course.

I trained as a supervisor first in the 1970s to work with social workers, and in the 1990s, following registration as a psychotherapist, I trained in transpersonal supervision. I first began supervising coaches while collaborating with two friends to co-create a coaching supervision course in 2005–06.

My coach training was initially with The Coaches Training Institute. I completed a Co-Active Coaching intermediate course, followed by an Insights Learning and Development programme. I then added HeartMath Practitioner Coach training (Heartmath, 2020), where I deepened my learning about and experience of the power of heart energy in relational coaching. My executive coaching and consulting experiences have been in both the public and private sectors.

Jane

I was born a fraternal twin in South Africa in 1962. I was educated at the University of the Witwatersrand, Johannesburg, where I graduated with a bachelor's degree in music and a postgraduate diploma in education. I continued studying through the University of South Africa, where I completed three years of psychology as an adjunct to my bachelor's degree. My working roles included teaching computer languages at a college and a six-year corporate stint as product manager for Technics Musical Instruments, a brand owned by Panasonic.

I emigrated to the United Kingdom in May 1999 and was granted British citizenship five years later. It was during this time that I made the decision to pursue a career in coaching, and in 2002 I enrolled in a one-year programme with the Coaching Academy to develop the necessary skills. Shortly thereafter, I joined forces with a fellow coach and entrepreneur, and we established a coaching company to support individuals and teams in organisations. Since then, I have had the good fortune to coach many individuals in both organisational settings and in their personal capacity.

My therapy training includes a foundation year in integrative psychotherapy at Metanoia, a diploma in stress management, an advanced certificate in cognitive-behavioural approaches to psychotherapy and counselling, an intensive six-month introduction to psychodynamic counselling and psychotherapy and, most recently, the first year of a master's degree in mindfulness-based psychotherapeutic practice at the Karuna Institute in Devon. I had hoped to finally complete a psychotherapeutic training here, following the aspirations I'd had since I was in my early thirties, but the circumstances of my life shaped a different decision.

In 2006, I began practising mindfulness in its intrapersonal form. In 2007, while attending a seven-day silent insight meditation retreat at Gaia House in Devon, I learned about Gregory Kramer's relational meditational practice of Insight Dialogue (ID) (Kramer, Meleo-Meyer, and Turner, 2008) and a year later attended my first ID retreat. Concurrently, I discovered the master's programme in mindfulness-based approaches at Bangor University's Centre for Mindfulness Research and Practice. I enrolled in the part-time course and graduated a few years later. My qualitative research project was devoted to the exploration of authenticity as both an intrapersonal and interpersonal phenomenon.

I taught Jon Kabat-Zinn's empirically validated Mindfulness-Based stress Reduction (MBSR) course for many years. I also had the opportunity to teach the Interpersonal Mindfulness course, an eight-week programme based on ID. In 2016, I added Kristen Neff and Christopher Germer's Mindful Self-Compassion eight-week programme (2018) to my teaching portfolio. In June that year, I completed a supervision training course through Bangor and since then have been offering supervision to mindfulness teachers, both privately and as an associate for The Mindfulness Network, a charity that works closely with Bangor University and other mindfulness-based interventions training organisations.

I have been delivering mindfulness to the corporate sector since 2011, and that remains a passion. Most recently, my interest has been in offering relational mindfulness interventions to foster psychological safety and humanise the workplace through the power of dialogical relationships.

Introduction to the developmental phases in our relationship

In our mutual transformational learning process, we attended to the two facets of adult learning concurrently: horizontal and vertical development. In adult learning for professional and personal development, both are important. During the first phase of our work together, the emphasis was more on horizontal growth, with the expansion of our personal and professional competencies and qualities. As our relationship deepened, we moved into the territory of vertical development, which supported a mutual evolution of our levels of consciousness, enhancing our capacity for complexity, ambiguity, and uncertainty.

The phases we identified in our work together were:

1 building the relationship with the known and the yet to be known about our relational capacities
2 taking our first steps towards attending to our vertical development through opening to our shared vulnerability
3 deepening resonant relational attunement through relational mindfulness practices that supported our emergent dialogue and a post-conventional consciousness.

Here we each share our evolutionary process, illustrated with key moments that enabled shifts in *how* we worked as we gradually moved towards an increasingly authentic, loving, and emergent dialogue that facilitated our reciprocal learning and development.

Phase 1: September 2006 to February 2008: Building the relationship with the known and the yet to be known about our relational capacities

Jane

Fiona and I began working together in early September 2006. Prior to this, I had little experience of supervision so I was a novice to this process.

At the end of our third session, in mid-November, I remember telling Fiona that I felt I could trust her. I was aware of her background as a transpersonal psychotherapist. Having had many years of personal therapy prior to 2006 I recognised the sense of safety that came from conferring this sub-role on Fiona. Her capacity to meet me with warm positive regard repeatedly sent messages to my nervous system that it was safe to be with this person. I started to take tentative steps towards bringing material that would expose my weaknesses, reveal blind spots, and offer growth opportunities.

Fiona

My focus in this early phase was to establish a working relationship with Jane. My choices and actions were based on being the expert and a warm and friendly tutor with a new supervisee.

I focused with Jane on developing an understanding of her experience of working with her clients. I looked at what might be going on and the concerns Jane had about her competency. I was reassured when Jane told me that she felt she could be real with me, to trust me. At this point we had developed a good rapport. Neither of us explored what this comment meant. This was reflective of and appropriate to the level of relational depth at this stage in our working together.

When Jane said she felt she could trust me, I thought to myself that I must have been doing something right. A hint here of my unconscious anxiety – would I be good enough to work with Jane when my supervision experience with executive coaches was still relatively new? I was also a novice. Reading my notes now brings home to me that although I was an experienced supervisor, I was not ready to acknowledge my anxiety about my competency as a coach supervisor because it held the potential for shame.

Jane

The themes that I explored in the sessions during this first phase of our working together were typical of a novice coach. They included: I must 'get it right'; I need to make a difference; self-doubt; and anxiety about my competency. I also brought many examples of interactions where I was taking too much responsibility for the client's growth through wanting to help or fix. I unpacked this and began to explore the associated anxieties and vulnerabilities around being good enough. This started to move us into more personal territory.

Up to this point in our work together, I was aware of regarding Fiona as the 'expert' and myself as the learner. Although in role terms this was accurate, this positioning is inherently unhelpful as it sets up an unhealthy imbalance of power in the relationship. Psychologically, this was a pattern of mine: to be deferential to people who I perceived were more knowledgeable than I was. This pattern also featured in interactions with people I regarded as highly intelligent, where I would feel intimidated and disempowered. These elements were a feature of my early relationship with Fiona.

Fiona

My response to Jane's concern about wanting to help people was to share my own version of this, which is one of my sub-personalities, who I call 'Helpful Harriet'. I disclosed that this part of me would appear when I felt stuck or concerned that I wasn't getting it right. Revealing this was my first step towards a more authentic way of being with myself and with Jane. I was beginning to work from behind my persona, rather than acting out with this part of my unconscious mind. However, I did not openly explore the deeper psychodynamics that triggered this sub-personality and the impact it had on our working relationship until later.

I can now see that I was familiar with and at ease with a tutorial style process. This was my conscious model of supervision, the seven-eyed model of Hawkins and Shohet (2012), with my focus on those 'eyes' that are about the supervisee's clients and her relationship with them, the interventions made, and Jane's concern to be a competent coach.

At this point in our work, I was on safe ground, schooled in models and theories, and generally on what I would call the received wisdom held in the supervision community, which places high value on evidence-based practice, and on cognitive, conceptual thinking – left brain explicit processes. This is the domain of knowing and certainty. I was not yet ready to move from this territory into more right brain embodied and implicit knowing processes, which by their very nature evoke uncertainty.

Driven by my anxiety, I had given Jane a list of my credentials at our first meeting. Much later, during phase 2 when I was sharing with my supervisor my delight at the deeper work I was doing with Jane, she said with a smile, 'Oh you were busy parading your wares at the start then, weren't you?' I said to her that she was spot on. I imagine that I came across as ready to teach Jane, setting the scene with my intention and focus for the working relationship from my perspective. Our verbal contract was simply a practical one concerning meetings and fees. Some years prior to undertaking this role, I had retired from academia and, on reflection, I realise I was unconsciously mourning the loss of a role and the status it had afforded me, and not yet quite ready to let go of elements of that role to leave space for a new way of being and working.

Phase 1: Learning reflections

This phase was characterised by a horizontal learning process, in part derived from the imbalance of power in our relationship with the assuming of and identification with the roles of supervisor as expert and supervisee as learner. We each had conscious and unconscious fears that took time to emerge fully and be talked about. Cognitive and analytic learning took a central place during this phase. We were both model and tools bound, seeking certainty.

What this means is that we were both inhabiting our prescribed roles and playing out socially learned and shaped behaviours relative to this context. We were doing 'the right thing' and being goal oriented. We were both also able to think abstractly and be self-reflective. However, as Kegan (1982) notes, at this stage we felt deferential and vulnerable to following what we thought we ought to be doing.

Phase 2: February 2008 to 2010: Opening up to our shared vulnerability, balancing the personal with the professional; first steps towards attending to our vertical development

Jane

I knew that Fiona's previous work was that of an academic, and I was intimidated by her considerable knowledge and expertise. Consequently, my learning style up to this point had largely been shaped and characterised by a fear of being seen as incompetent. I adopted more of a defensive strategy, both unconsciously and consciously, in my relationship with her. Self-critical thoughts and editing of what I chose to share inhibited real relational contact and the capacity to be open to learning at depth.

During one session, 'Helpful Harriet' emerged and I fell into the incompetency hole. I was triggered into the not-good-enough pattern where I felt disempowered, small, and filled with self-doubt and shame. At that moment, I made the decision to take a risk. I shared with Fiona how I was feeling as I could see it was interfering with my learning process. I remember how vulnerable I felt as I named it. My heart was pounding. The childhood expectation that I'd be judged and rejected followed in the wake of this self-disclosure. Surprisingly, Fiona reciprocated and openly disclosed her own vulnerability.

Fiona

I felt immediately taken aback and yet touched by Jane's courage in declaring her feelings in this way. I acknowledged that I too was having doubts about my competency. I shared elements of my experience of feeling I had no value unless I came across as knowing what I was talking about and being helpful. During this early phase of our working together, when I was held in my conventional, survival mode of thinking, 'Helpful Harriet' would appear unbidden at times, primed and ready to help, to fix and to be seen as having value.

Learning reflections

We recognised that we had entered an unconscious, mutually created dance. Unwittingly, our relationship was retriggering and reinforcing our unconscious childhood wounds associated with not being good enough. We had been completely ensnared in this stress-inducing relational pattern until I, Jane, had the courage to be vulnerable and shared my feelings of incompetence in relation to Fiona. It was now out in the open, accessible to the healing light of our mutual awareness.

Much of our dialogue about our fear of being seen as incompetent felt deeply reassuring to us, in that we could learn together, and be open about what was happening within us and in our relational field. The sharing we did that day changed the course of our working relationship and moved us closer to reciprocal learning. We both felt we were in the process of releasing our mutual fear of not being good enough, which had held us back.

We emerged from previously held quite fixed roles, developed a deeper trust in the process and in each other, and took a step towards greater acceptance of our vulnerability as well as our strengths. We could both see also that the power dynamic in which we had been operating had begun to equalise through our mutual willingness to be relationally authentic. Compassion for our shared human predicament began to flow.

Jane

In my second year of the Bangor University master's degree, I decided to take the Mindfulness and Individual Therapy module. The university agreed to Fiona taking on the role of my supervisor during this time. What was interesting for me was that I started to flex and deepen our relationship through broadening the context of our work together. Working in a different context brought up different material. It was during this time that I frequently expressed concern regarding the boundary between coaching and therapy, a common inquiry for many coaches. Even though I had spent years in personal therapy and studied psychotherapy, I questioned whether I had the necessary skills to be able to discern how far into the therapeutic territory was appropriate in coaching.

I also explored the application of mindfulness in the coaching process. At this stage, mindfulness featured more implicitly in how I was attending to my clients and what I noticed in my own process. This included the territory of transference and counter-transference, how this is felt and known in the body and mind, and how it shapes behavioural impulses.

What strikes me about the preparation I did at that time, as reflected in my emails to Fiona, was that there was a lot of detail. I did a careful analysis, working things out before talking with her. This was associated with the need to be well prepared, to be sure of what I was saying before our meeting. Although I had moved forward significantly regarding our level of trust, it still felt too risky and unsafe to lean into the inherent uncertainty of the present moment, feel into the body and open to the learning emerging from this embodied and relationally generative place. At this stage I had been practising relational mindfulness in the form of Insight Dialogue for just over a year. My conceptual understanding of opening to and listening from the body to connect with emergent wisdom was growing; however, it took a few years before I could embody this understanding in relationship.

Fiona

During this new phase, as I read Jane's emails, I felt drawn into my former academic tutor role once again, to join with her Bangor tutors. It was as if in this new context I felt a need to change our established way of relating and find a new way. Now I recognise that there was anxiety in our relational field evoked by this new task, and we were both resonating with it.

I recorded in my notes: 'Jane tells me she is fearful of straying into territory that she is not fully trained for.' A session that exemplifies this was when her client shared that she felt unable to trust people. In her work with Jane, she shared that she was beginning to feel safe in their relationship. Jane described that she stayed with and explored her client's feelings and fears, working developmentally rather than behaviourally. I had often seen Jane's capacity to work therapeutically with some clients, and reassured her that she was remaining within her capacities.

I had been concerned about the issue of the boundary between coaching and therapy, notwithstanding the differences in terms of tasks and agendas, and especially of holding back on my own view that there is a considerable overlap in terms of meta skills. For us, the real discussion here is what is going to work, and whether the coach is knowledgeable and skilful enough, rather than describing the boundaries and seeing these accounts as prescriptive. I reflected on the importance of embodied relational learning as one of the keys to effective change in both coaching and therapy.

Our supervision on the module brought a fuller focus on relational mindfulness into our dialogues.

Jane and I noticed that I had been too reassuring and not attended to her anxieties enough. I recall that while I was aware of my shallow breathing and tension in my shoulders as Jane described her concerns about her competency, I did not share my somatic experience. I missed this opportunity because I was once again caught up in my need to be helpful.

I was unconsciously moved to reassure Jane about what she was doing rather than exploring her anxieties. For a time, we dropped back into the mutual process that reinforced our fears of being seen as incompetent – the dance of our two nervous systems. I appreciate that it takes many conscious iterations before deeply rooted defensive relational patterns can be healed.

Jane

Since 2002, I had the good fortune to be in a business partnership with a highly talented and charismatic man. Our partnership was successful for many years and our mutual collaborative learning was rich. As a result of the deepening of my meditation practice and my master's studies, I recognised that I wanted to go in a different direction and we started to have conversations around ending our work together.

It was during this turbulent time that I asked Fiona whether she would be willing to take on the role of my coach for a few months, to support me to take the necessary steps towards leaving the partnership. We re-contracted around this, establishing the new boundaries for our work together. The material I brought to the sessions became much more personal. This served to once again broaden the context within which we were working together, and it also afforded us both the opportunity to see and experience each other differently. When we emerged out of this phase of our working together, re-contracting for supervision once again, our relationship had become more resilient, trust had been fortified, and we were on different ground. My supervision notes began to reflect a deeper openness and vulnerability. I felt more comfortable to name my inadequacies and speak about experiences where I felt shame.

Fiona

I had noted some weeks earlier that Jane's business relationship was not working well for her and the 'Helpful Harriet' part of me wanted to help her to 'just leave now!' as I had had a similar experience myself. Once I realised that I had been triggered and was over-identified with Jane's story, I shared this with her, owning that it was hard for me to remain neutral. I was then able to get out of my own way to support her more fully to work through the challenges and to arrive at a place of greater clarity.

Jane

During this time, I was just beginning to experiment with taking mindfulness into the workplace, and I was invited to give a three-hour taster workshop for a company called Enthum in Lewes, East Sussex. I invited Fiona to attend this session. I remember feeling somewhat uncomfortable and a little uncertain as I related to her as a member of the group. Although the formal roles of supervisor and supervisee had loosened considerably over the four years we had known each other, this was the first step towards a more collegiate relationship.

Fiona

I loved reversing our roles when I attended the Enthum workshop on Mindful Leadership held by Jane. When I saw Jane in this new context, I had an opportunity to see different facets of her, to learn more about her.

I had not seen Jane in person for at least a year, as we had worked on the telephone for months before then and only more recently virtually via Skype and then Zoom. When I saw her – not just her head and shoulders – I spontaneously remarked, 'Oh you have become a woman!' I thought afterwards what an extraordinary thing I had blurted out. This exclamation was an expression of cognitive dissonance. In other words, my previous unconscious perception of Jane was incongruent with what I was consciously seeing at that moment. She came across as a woman of authority and presence, who I thought ran a creative workshop in an engaging way. At our first meeting, I saw Jane as an anxious young student needing my help. There I could see that while our relational dance had begun between 'Helpful Harriett', my mothering/tutoring self, and Jane's needy child self, our relationship had changed. Our co-created pattern had exemplified our early way of relating. The context in which I saw Jane that day, as well as in the workshop process itself, brought about a big shift in our relationship. I saw her as a colleague with whom I could learn even more now, not just within our supervision relationship.

I noticed that in much of my work with Jane, especially as a supervisor with others, I was becoming freer to work relationally. I noticed that I was sensing as much in my body as in my thinking what was going on in the dialogue, moment by moment, and dipping in and out of different facets of the process. I was becoming more playful at times too – for example, as in the comment to Jane when I first saw her at the Enthum workshop. I was not trying to be 'a supervisor', but rather being fully myself, sharing spontaneously how I perceived Jane at that moment.

I was shifting my consciousness of Jane, still in supervision with me and now a colleague in the business of facilitation and the development of coaches. It felt to me that the relationship was now collegial, and that it reflected the steps we were making on our vertical development. I felt myself shifting beyond my socialised mind, from being tied to a way of practice learned from imbibing tools and models towards a more self-authoring stage. I also noticed qualities emerging that are associated with a self-transforming mind, where I was becoming open to a more dialogical, emergent way of being. I was consciously drawing on the transformational learning paradigm (Gergen, 2009; Garvey Berger, 2012; Kegan, 2009).

I was finding it very liberating to discover that while I could draw on what I had learned cognitively about how to 'do' supervision, these relational experiences had been as great a teacher about how to 'be' a supervisor as anything I had read or even learned on a course!

Phase learning reflections

We recognised that we were beginning to let go of prescribed roles of teacher and learner and were becoming more fluid in how we worked together in the here and now. We were also challenging some conventional views about what supervision is, especially ways that are solely models-based and tools-based, and that maintained a power imbalance as the way to work.

Phase 3: 2011 to present: Deeper resonant relational attunement through relational mindfulness practices that support emergent dialogue and post-conventional consciousness

Jane

In February 2011, at the age of 47, I fell pregnant for the first time. The circumstances surrounding the pregnancy were challenging and there were too many health risks associated with carrying a child at my age, for the baby and myself. It was therefore not possible to go through with the pregnancy. This was one of the most difficult periods of my life, as I mourned the loss of the baby and the possibility of being a mother. I shared this with Fiona during one of our sessions. Her response touched me deeply, as it took us into tender mutual territory.

Fiona

I burst into tears on hearing this news, and shared what it had evoked for me. I felt an immediate sense that I was not being judged but rather simply held compassionately in Jane's presence. It was such a poignant moment. I later explored this moment more fully in my own supervision as it had affected me very deeply, particularly my grief at not having had children of my own. With my supervisor's full loving acceptance of my tears, we reflected on what else might have been triggered. Some years ago, my mother had shared with me that she had been very anxious and distressed when she discovered she was pregnant after my father had just left to join the 8th army in North Africa. Had she felt she could not bear being pregnant, and had her feelings been communicated to my twin and I before we were born? Jane's pregnancy certainly stirred up a great deal of emotion that had been buried very deeply until triggered in that moment. I learned that day that as supervisors it is important for our supervisee's wellbeing that we can hold an open and loving space for what may happen in supervision relationships that reveal our authentic selves. We all carry experiences that hold energy that may not have emerged into consciousness. Once acknowledged, our energy is then freed to be available for the present tasks in which we are engaged.

I recognised I could risk being real in this relationship and receive a loving response. I experienced no self-criticism regarding my self-disclosure; rather, it was simply what happened in the moment. Formerly, I might have chastised myself for how I responded. I started to recognise that I was becoming compassionate towards myself. Having said that, I do realise now that I am still fearful of being judged by some of my colleagues about revealing my vulnerability in this way.

Jane

In 2013, I trained to teach the Interpersonal Mindfulness eight-week programme, the secular offering based on Kramer's Insight Dialogue practice (Kramer, Meleo-Meyer, and Turner, 2008). I mentioned to Fiona that I was running a course in London and invited her to attend as a full participant. I so wanted her to have the opportunity to experience this profound practice. I also felt it would add further depth to our work together and enhance our capacity to work in a more embodied way, attune more sensitively to the relational field, and open ourselves to the emergent wisdom therein.

Once again, it was so interesting to take on the role of 'teacher' in relation to Fiona; however, this time it was on a much deeper and more actively engaged level. I had the opportunity to observe her in mindful dialogue with course participants and at times engaged with her in an inquiry process, exploring what she noticed during the practices. This afforded me the opportunity to see Fiona in an entirely different light. I saw her vulnerability more clearly and recognised her very human limitations. This was a significant milestone in the maturation of our relationship. The remnants of her role as 'expert' were dissolved into love through compassion for our shared human imperfection. It was very moving for me.

My supervision notes reflected the changes that had occurred in our learning relationship. I was willing to show Fiona my 'true imperfect self'. Recognising that there was no right or wrong, I felt more comfortable to explore my ideas more fully. Significantly, I trusted that I was not going to be shamed for sharing my ideas. This also supported me to be much clearer about what I needed from our time together and more specifically what I needed from Fiona as my supervisor.

Fiona

I loved being a student on Jane's course. I experienced her wisdom and compassion for the group as we were all learning together to stay mindfully present in our dialogues. Although I had been practising meditation for many years and had been drawn to a Buddhist perspective on life, here I learned to bring mindfulness directly into being relationally present, in body and in mind. This was an eye opener. In the practice sessions, I particularly learned at a bodily level some of the ways I was triggered at times to want to fix my partner's difficulties, get into therapy mode, and distract myself from being fully present. I developed greater insight into my relational patterns and felt increasingly compassionate towards myself and members of the group. I felt truly seen, felt, and accepted in all my humanness. As I write these words, I feel tearful, recognising how much I had longed for this kind of acceptance.

This experience built on the earlier one of being a participant in Jane's Enthum workshop. I was seeing her again as a very experienced facilitator and coach. On this occasion, I knew that could learn more about myself in relationships, not just from our supervision relationship but also my relational styles, personally as well as professionally. During some of the dialogues, I saw again my 'Helpful Harriet' being embodied as I felt myself leaning forward slightly into the space between myself and my partner. I was able to notice somatically and then restore my ground without getting involved.

The whole ethos of the course was to be a compassionate witness to our own process, to hold our humanity tenderly. I have since consciously brought this ethos into my own life, and often introduce it into my work with clients when I sense they are becoming very self-critical. I would have said of myself that I was compassionate and non-judgemental, yet this experience brought home to me the difference between what I espoused and what I could consciously choose to be like in action. I knew that from then on I may well be triggered into reactivity, yet now with more capacity to notice without judgement and to set a new course in the next few moments.

I think that the best way I can describe the effect this experience had on me and how I related to Jane was that I no longer identified with the role of expert, consciously or unconsciously. From that point on, I felt free to offer my expertise and engage with whatever arose within me and between us. It felt like we were both free to flow – or not – together. If there had been any vestige of pressure remaining in me to 'get it right as a supervisor', that had completely gone.

This new sense of my way of being, having expertise but not holding the role of expert, has transformed my work as a coach and supervisor. Since then, I have been working in this way with all my supervisees. I use myself as an instrument (Bachkirova, 2016) in my work, where I bring my capacity to stay in an emergent dialogue and respond from that place.

I feel a great debt of gratitude that our relationship of mutual learning and healing has enabled me to come to a deep sense of my real self, body, mind, and spirit, with all my strengths as well as acceptance of my frailties. I love my work as a supervisor and feel great joy at discovering that whatever trips me up as I endeavour to stay alongside folk, I have the capacity to recover from wobbles and get back in step. Working with Jane enabled me to step away from feeling responsible for her learning and to facilitate her own inner wisdom, while sharing my own when invited to do so.

Final reflections from us both

Our work together has evolved into a relationally attuned and loving learning partnership. Our mutual appreciation and practice of relational mindfulness opened our dialogues to the nuances of how we related to one another, as well as to their content. We are comfortable to be authentic with each other, to reveal our uncertainties, to meet our shared vulnerability without judgement. We have developed emotionally through our capacity to attune to one another and to access a kind of knowing that comes from how it feels to be with this person at this moment in time (Tronick et al., 1977). Siegel's (2010) term for the capacity to attune in this way is a 'mindsight skill'.

Our listening for each other is enriched. We have developed a deeper layer of processing through the nature of our embodied inquiry by letting go of analysing and rather being more present to the body and to what is emerging here now. We can stay with discomfort in the body rather than react to it, and are able to bring our discomfort into the dialogue as data to explore. Consequently, we recognised that our dialogues are occurring at a much slower pace. The sessions are more spacious, and silences are more available – the impulse to fill the space has quietened. Our nervous systems are settled, which facilitates creative thinking. We are also much more spontaneous and able to laugh at our idiosyncrasies and very human weaknesses. All this is testimony to the high degree of mutual safety that we co-created over the years of our working together. Ultimately, we have supported each other's growth as human beings. We discovered together what it is was like 'if we approached one another through love, with delight and pleasure' Wheatley (1998: 1).

Summary

In this chapter, we have charted the development of our supervision relationship over a period of 12 years. We explored how our evolving mindfulness-based relational process facilitated transformational learning and new ways of being for both of us. We explored how the deepening sense of safety enabled us to reveal our human vulnerabilities and that this matured into mutual love and compassionate presence, enhancing our reflective capacities and learning.

Questions for reflection

1 Were there any moments during your reading of our case study where you felt uncomfortable and/or critical of either Fiona or Jane? Did this reveal something regarding your preferred way of working with your clients?
2 In reflecting on a session, are there times where you have felt you should have done something differently? Perhaps you experienced some self-judgement or even shame?
3 Do you have a sense about what role you are most comfortable inhabiting in your supervision or coaching relationships?
4 At what moment in a supervision or coaching conversation might you consider sharing something personal?
5 Do you have a sense that your client relationships are evolving? If yes, what are you noticing that would suggest this?

References

Bachkirova, T. (2016). The Self of the Coach: Conceptualization Issues, and Opportunities for Practitioner Development. *Consulting Psychology Journal: Practice and Research, 68*(2), 143–56.

Garvey Berger, J. (2012). *Changing on the Job: Developing Leaders for a Complex World.* Stanford, CA: Stanford University Press.
Gergen, K. (2009). *Relational Being: Beyond Self and Community.* New York: Oxford University Press.
Hawkins, P. and Shohet, R. (2012). *Supervision in the Helping Professions.* Maidenhead: Open University Press.
Heartmath Institute (2020). *Coach Training Course for Certified and Licensed HeartMath Practitioner.* www.heartmath.org (accessed 20 February 2021).
Kegan, R. (1982). *The Evolving Self: Problem and Process in Human Development.* Cambridge, MA: Harvard University Press.
Kegan, R. and Lahey, L. (2009). *Immunity to Change: How to Overcome It and Unlock the Potential in Yourself and Your Organization (Leadership for the Common Good).* San Francisco: Jossey-Bass.
Kramer, G., Meleo-Meyer, F., and Turner, M. L. (2008). Cultivating Mindfulness in Relationship Insight Dialogue and the Interpersonal Mindfulness Programme. In S. F. Hick, and T. Bien (eds), *Mindfulness and the Therapeutic Relationship.* New York: Guilford Press.
Neff, K. and Germer, C. (2018). *The Mindful Self-Compassion Workbook.* London: Guilford Press.
Siegel, D. (2010). *Mindsight: Transform Your Brain with the New Science of Kindness.* Oxford: One World.
Tronick, E., Als, H., and Adamson, L. (1977). The Structure of Face-to-Face Communicative Interactions. In M. Bullowa (ed.), *Before Speech.* Cambridge: Cambridge University Press, pp. 249–371.
Wheatley, M. (1998). Love and Fear in Organisations. *National Association of Student Personnel Administrators Newsletter, 20*(5), http://margaretwheatley.com/articles/love.html (accessed 20 February 2021).

Chapter 5

Meta-perspective on our learning journey

The Space Between Us

We awaken to this moment
the sights, the sounds
the gift of now:

this flow of breath
this beating heart
this skin that tingles

We scan for tensions
release each one
slip back into the flow

Sitting before you
the space between us
resonates with being

We open our hearts
trusting in a world
where all are one

Touched by humility
we let go of agendas
accept not-knowing

We see, listen deeply
as we speak our truth.
Memories shift

DOI: 10.4324/9781315161280-5

old certainties fray
time-served narratives
lose their grip

At last we're free
to re-shape our stories
find new ways to be
Henry Campion,
unpublished, 2021

Introduction

The three phases we reflected on in our case study in Chapter 4 charted the development of our supervision relationship. We described two intertwined facets of relating: one reflecting two human beings with their unique capacities, personal histories, and attachment styles; the other showing two coaching professionals in the business of being in a supervision relationship. Neither of us could have anticipated that we would co-create the necessary conditions for transformation to occur in our capacity to learn and how we were being in relationship with each other and with our clients.

Following the completion of our case study, we met frequently to dialogue about our process. The questions we were holding were these: What were the factors that contributed to our learning? What were the necessary conditions for our learning to be together fully and deeply in relationship? What was going on both within us and in the space between us? How did mindfulness influence our learning and transformation? We also reflected on what each of us brought to our growth process, and Chapter 3 is our response to this.

Our inquiry helped us to formulate a meta-perspective of our learning journey where we identified the meta skills, attitudes, qualities, and processes that facilitated our shift from a conventional relationship to a post-conventional dialogical relationship. It is clear to us that mindfulness was the transforming agent, in that it created the necessary conditions for relational depth.

Here we offer you the fruits of our reflective dialogues, beginning with distinguishing conventional relating from dialogical relating.

Conventional relating: subject-to-object

Martin Buber said all real living is meeting (Owen, 2018). At the most fundamental level, our human existence is relational. We need to be confirmed by others – attended to, accepted, acknowledged, respected, and loved. This enables us to be more grounded in a sense of our own existence, our authentic self, and to meet our deepest existential need: to be who we are.

Confirmation is so essential that if we don't receive it for being who we are, we will try to get it by appearing the way we think someone else would like us to be as an attempt to be loved. And we lose touch with our true self. This is the psychological wounding that underpins fear-based attachment styles. It is also the foundation of conventional levels of self-development where worry about what other people think about us shapes our behaviour.

The first phase of our supervision relationship was characterised by qualities of the socialised or conventional mind, where there is a subject-to-object relatedness that creates separateness and adherence to learned role behaviours. With our fear-based attachment styles, our capacity to trust was impaired. We didn't feel safe with each other or with ourselves. We operated from our false selves, each of us caught up in our own subjective experience, and objectified each other to better handle our anxiety and our existential frailty.

During the first years of working together, our relationship fitted the conventional supervisor–supervisee dynamic. The primary relational focus was all about establishing psychological safety as the foundation for the exploration and discovery that was essential to learning. The learning process requires that we can trust enough to step out of that which is known to us, that which feels secure, and take risks. Learning is dependent on the person's capacity for discomfort, and therefore the degree of learning is relative to the degree of safety in the relationship: if I don't feel safe, I can't be vulnerable and show myself. Fiona provided a safe holding environment for Jane's learning in that she attended to Jane's psychological needs to be seen, heard, accepted, acknowledged, and respected. Over time, Jane felt she could trust Fiona, and this enhanced her learning.

The key piece here is that the psychological safety was a unidirectional process. Fiona's human needs for the same were bracketed. Instead of finding safety in the relationship, Fiona stayed within the boundary of her role as an expert and the security provided by models and theories. Hycner (1991) refers to this as 'professional superiority'. She had established a rapport with Jane, and felt empathy and warmth for her; however, the meeting was partial.

Dialogical relating: subject-to-subject

The developmental trajectory of our work together changed when Jane took a risk and revealed her vulnerability. Fiona responded by reciprocating Jane's openness. This was the first step towards a post-conventional way of relating, predicated on the relational principle that genuine openness to others elicits a reciprocal response. Given that learning cannot be separated from relationship, this opened the space for mutual transformational learning to occur.

During the later phases of our working together, our relationship evolved into greater mutuality as we revealed more of our common humanity. Hycner, a dialogical psychotherapist, suggests that humanity has become equated with individuality, particularly in the Western social context. He proposes that 'our pursuing our *self* is not an end in itself, but rather our self is discovered and fulfilled in our relatedness to others' (Hycner, 1993: 78). True meeting in dialogue occurs when the practitioner (supervisor) is available to the supervisee, first as a human being and second as a professional trained in appropriate methods (Hycner, 1993). This applies equally to the supervisee. We came into a more equal relationship while inhabiting our respective roles lightly. We were able to rest in the paradoxical interdependent reality of separateness and relatedness, of individuality and relationality, characteristic of a dialogical relationship.

Trust was now mutual: we both felt safe enough with each other to reveal more of our vulnerabilities and be real in our relating. In essence, we were meeting each other's psychological needs to be seen, heard, accepted, acknowledged, and respected. There is another key facet in mutuality, which is trust in ourselves – building a safe and secure-base relationship to ourselves and our inner world. Jane's initial risk-taking required sufficient trust in the relationship *and* in herself. Whatever the consequences of her personal disclosure – Fiona's possible reactivity and defensiveness or reciprocal openness and responsiveness – she would be able to contain and process the emotions that arose.

Elements that evolved our relationship

Being in dialogue required an intention to engage in a particular kind of conversation that asked a great deal of us: taking the risk of openness to being changed as a person. Here we are talking about changes at both implicit and explicit levels of knowing, and where we are interacting rather than intervening (in the professional jargon), so we are each available to the other as learning partners, being open to changing ourselves as persons through dialogue. We increasingly brought more of our authentic selves into our meetings. Our experience of being authentic is that it is a shifting state rather than an immutable sense of self. Ibarra (2015) sees authenticity more as our learning to experiment with our identity, so it becomes related to who we are in the moment, rather than a state we can be in all the time. This conceptualisation of self is congruent with post-conventional ways of perceiving the self, as explored in Chapter 2.

Through our supervisor–supervisee experiences, we were able to identify many of the emergent characteristics inherent in dialogical relationships. These include:

- *Self-awareness and other awareness.* The capacity to use ourselves as an instrument for awareness is founded on an attitudinal stance of curiosity and openness in relation to ourselves and each other. What parts of me show up when I am with this person? What is the felt sense of being in this relationship? Where am I holding back? What am I fearful of? What has been triggered in me now? What might the discomfort I'm feeling in my body now reveal if I open myself to it? What might be revealed about each of us as the dialogue unfolds? What's here now in the field between us to be known?
- *Mutual vulnerability and honesty.* These qualities sit at the heart of dialogical relating. When we could be open to our fallibility and speak authentically from this place, we gave each other 'permission' to be human: we came out from behind the protective mask of the false self and our nervous systems co-regulated, relaxing as we entered the field of intersubjective vulnerability. These are the dialogical moments that foster growth, development, and authenticity within the intersubjective encounter (Gergen, 2009; Stolorow and Atwood, 1992). We learned to appreciate the paradoxical truth that vulnerability is a strength rather than a weakness, which we both had been socially conditioned to believe. Brené Brown (2010) describes vulnerability as the core of meaningful relational experiences. She asserts that it is the birthplace of love, belonging, joy, courage, empathy, and creativity, and also the source of hope, empathy, accountability, and authenticity.

- *Speaking the truth.* Having the courage to be vulnerable is inextricably linked to the capacity to speak the truth of one's subjective experience in the moment.
- *Adopting a growth mindset.* It is necessary to face the paradox of being comfortable with discomfort and seeing discomfort as an essential part of growth.
- *Seeing failure through the lens of a growth mindset.* With our fear-based attachment styles, we both had the propensity to regard failure as something personal, believing it had to do with our own sense of inadequacy, of not being good enough. Furthermore, our social conditioning established a link between failure and fear, a common construct in Western educational systems. In our work together, we moved to a place where we could be curious about our experiences of failure and what they could teach us. Pema Chodron gave a commencement address to the 2014 graduating class of Naropa University in Boulder, Colorado. She couched failure in these terms: 'Try again. Fail again. Fail better.'

  > This illustrates an attitudinal shift that is essential for growth: 'If you want to be a full, complete human being, if you want to be genuine and not pretend that everything is either one way or the other way but you can hold the fullness of life in your heart, then this is the opportunity to get curious about what is going on and listen to the storylines. And you don't buy the ones that blame it on everybody else. And you don't buy the storylines that blame it on yourself, either'.
  >
  > (Chodron, 2015: 66)

  As our relationship evolved, our ideas about failure changed. We moved from the conventional dualistic failure–success, right–wrong conceptualisation to a compassionate stance where we recognised the interdependence of many factors shaping our capacity to respond skilfully in the moment. A Rumi quote captures the essence of this in his poem 'A Great Wagon': 'Out beyond ideas of wrongdoing and rightdoing there is a field. I'll meet you there. When the soul lies down in that grass the world is too full to talk about' (Rumi, 1995: 35; see also Barks, 1995).
- *Making choices aligned with our personal values*, rather than conforming to a socially conditioned prescriptive way of doing things.

- *Appropriate mutual disclosure.* Many of the transformational moments of our journey were shaped by our willingness to share our relevant life experiences in service of deepening the learning. In these moments – many of which were poignant – we met in the common ground of our humanity, outside our respective roles. This was one of the factors that helped to loosen our identification with these 'transactional' roles. Linked to this, the boundaries relating to what was appropriate and what was not appropriate to bring to the session became relaxed. We moved from fixed rules or ideas to an openness to the fluidity of emergence, to the here now, and trusted in the relevance of this.
- *Welcoming conflict.* We both welcomed conflict, regarding it as an agent for our mutual growth and development.
- *The capacity for mature empathic attunement.* Essentially, empathy is the ability to sense other people's emotions, coupled with the ability to imagine what someone else might be thinking or feeling. With the socialised mind, an experience of empathy typically triggers the desire to help the other and offer unsolicited advice to try to change or fix them. This is frequently an unconscious aversive response to feeling the pain of the other. It often results in a shift in power, where the one offering the advice takes on the role of the expert, imposing their take on reality as the 'right way'. There is no mutuality here. In the early days of our work, Fiona's 'Helpful Harriet' part was triggered in response to Jane's feelings of inadequacy. Her expertise became mobilised to 'make things better' for Jane, thereby easing her own anxiety. Similarly, Jane's early work with her clients clearly exhibited more of a reactive empathy, where she followed unconscious impulses to help or fix her clients. Experiencing empathy post-conventionally is quite different. In moments of true dialogue, advice-giving falls away and it is possible to be with the other where they are, respecting that they have their own journey and frame of reference. This is the essence of equanimous listening and is the soil for giving and receiving, of mutual growth.
- *The skill of adjusting from mis-attunement through disruption to reattunement.* As humans, we move in and out of connection with ourselves and others all the time. Perhaps the most central of relational skills is the capacity to move through the discomfort of a triggered nervous system back into regulation, both personally and interpersonally. This deepens self and other awareness, relational intimacy, and compassion. Without the

ability to regulate, we can get lost in blame stories, defensive states, and painful emotions. This will have an impact on our ability to learn and grow. We have learned that it is so important to notice that we have been triggered into reactivity and to name it. This act of courage and generosity offers material in service of learning and development for us both.

- *The ability to own our strengths and weaknesses with humility and humour.* This opens the possibility for play and fun in the relationship. It offers an opportunity to let go of doing and arrive in a state of being together. This facilitates a deepening of connection and cultivates healing. Play is the purest expression of love, as pointed out by author and psychiatrist Stuart Brown (2009).
- *Negative capability.* This is the ability to let go of the need to control, the need to find resolution or answers and to sit in silence, opening to the uncertainty inherent in the present moment. The phrase 'negative capability' was first used by Keats (2009) in 1817. Resting in this expansiveness allows room for a deeper listening to happen. This offers a gateway into the dynamic flow of information in the relational field. Thoughts, emotions, intuitions, and insights can arise from this place. It is here that true meeting arises.
- *Negative relational capability.* This is the ability to let go of the certainty created through concepts and ideas *about* the person you are with – for example, their personality style, their history, failings, and strengths – and instead meet them in the emergent field of 'not knowing'. What is showing up now in this person? Who are they being right now? What is here now in this co-created field? Groves (2016) describes this as being empty of concepts about the person sitting in front of you. This offers entry into a liminal space, a place of transformation: 'When behind you lies all that is known, and you stand on the threshold of the unknown to which the process of change leads you … What I want and intend to say is changed by the impact of hearing myself speak and your response to what I say. My will, which led me to initiate the dialogue, surrenders to the grace and intentionality of the emerging conversation' (Denham-Vaughan, 2010: 38).
- *Somatic awareness.* This is the ability to be present and connected to the body, feeling the feet on the floor, the bottom in the chair, poised, in the present moment. Through being connected to the body, we can more easily recognise when we

> have been triggered into relational reactivity. There is greater capacity to pause, notice, and then make a conscious choice about how best to respond to what is here. The body is also the gateway to the transpersonal, the intersubjective field that holds the relational consciousness.

Beyond subject-to-subject: the transpersonal intersubjective field

Transformation took place in our intersubjective field, the 'between', this system of mutual reciprocal influence. This field is a living dynamic medium where what arose and was noticed between us arose interdependently (Hargaden, 2015). It contained the conscious and unconscious material of us both. Mindful presence enabled us to access this field through quietening our analytical thinking minds and connecting us to our bodies, the anchor in the present moment. This opened the door to the field and intuitive wisdom with a shift in emphasis from our left-brain oriented language-based conceptual knowing to more of a right-brain embodied intuitive knowing (Woods, 2009). The pace of our dialogue slowed right down naturally to give spaces for what could come into our consciousness. As we listened deeply to our bodies, we learned to allow our bodies to speak. We gradually became open to what we were sensing as we sat together, face to face or virtually, vulnerable and open to whatever was arising.

Almaas and Johnson (2013) suggest that the more mature we are – that is, the less reactive and caught up in the narratives of the past – the more the relational field can deepen and expand and open to new potential.

Love lies at the heart of learning

> I've come to realise that on those rare occasions where we are fully met by another; when we are both truly seen and understood, the illusion of separation disappears and love is all that remains.
>
> (Shohet and Shohet, 2020: 20)

Through our work together, we reached a place where we recognised that the key ingredient in transformational learning is, in essence, love. Love blossomed in our relational moments of openness and vulnerability as we deepened into mutuality. Mutuality is the essence of mature love and authentic connection – being sensitive to the being we are with while being true to our authentic self. We feel both separate and yet deeply connected, profoundly nourished by those moments when our separateness dissolves, and we are liberated from fear.

By becoming free over time to work mindfully and lovingly, we can stay in our relationship at times of uncertainty, and especially in those very human moments when we are triggered and become reactive. Writing about love in counselling Suzanne Keys says, 'Love is not only about warmth, flow and close connection but also about being committed to the process of relating, with all its disconnections' (Keys, 2017: 35). Being in our co-created learning partnership was, and continues to be, an emotional undertaking, and love is what enables our relational experience to be authentic, curious, playful, and creative.

Conclusion

We came to experience that the mind is inherently embodied, social, interpersonal, and interactional. This is a key rationale for a relational model of supervision and coaching. Mindfulness, as an intrapersonal and interpersonal process, formed the bedrock of our work together. Through being present for ourselves and each other, we learned to co-create the optimal conditions for reciprocal learning, and this has transformed – and continues to transform – us both. We now see supervision as a spiritual practice, and our dialogues are love and compassion in action.

Summary

In this chapter, we have offered up the fruits of our reflective dialogues, where we formulated a meta-perspective of our learning journey. We explored what it means to shift from a conventional subject–object relationship to a post-conventional subject-to-subject relationship. We identified the meta skills, attitudes, qualities, and processes that we emergently discovered in our dialogical process. We also explored the transpersonal phenomenon of the relational field, a living dynamic medium that is more than the sum of the parts. Finally, we shared our recognition that love is the key ingredient in transformational learning, and that mutuality is the essence of mature love and authentic connection. We can live in the paradox of being sensitive and open to the person we are with *and* be true to our authentic self.

Questions for reflection

1 Which of the qualities of dialogical relationships resonates most strongly for you in terms of your experience in your coaching and supervision?
2 Similarly, which quality or qualities feel like learning edges?
3 What does risk-taking in your professional relationships mean to you?
4 How might you introduce creative play into your relational work?

References

Almaas, A. H. and Johnson, K. (2013). *The Power of Divine Eros: The Illuminating Force of Love in Everyday Life.* Boston: Shambala.

Barks, C. (1995). *The Essential Rumi.* San Francisco: Harper.

Brown, B. (2010). *The Gifts of Imperfection.* Harmondsworth: Penguin.

Brown, S. (2009). *Play: How It Shapes the Brain, Opens the Imagination, and Invigorates the Soul.* New York: Penguin.

Chodron, P. (2015). *Fail, Fail Again, Fail Better: Wise advice for Leaning into the Unknown.* Boulder, CO: Sounds True.

Denham-Vaughan, S. (2010). The Liminal Space and Twelve Action Practices for Gracious Living. *British Gestalt Journal, 19*(2), 34–45.

Gergen, K. (2009). *Relational Being: Beyond Self and Community.* New York: Oxford University Press.

Groves, S. (2016). *Presence in Relationship: Offering Core Process Psychotherapy.* Scotts Valley, CA: Create Space.

Hargaden, H. (ed.) (2015). *The Art of Relational Supervision: Clinical Implications of the Use of Self in Group Supervision.* London: Taylor and Francis.

Hycner, R. (1993) *Between Person and Person: Toward a Dialogical Psychotherapy.* Goldsboro, ME: Gestalt Journal Press.

Ibarra, H. (2015) *Act Like a Leader, Think Like a Leader.* Brighton, MA: Harvard Business Review Press.

Keats, J. (2009 [1817]). From a Letter to His Brothers. In O. Li (ed.), *Keats and Negative Capability.* London: Continuum, p. ix.

Keys, S. (2017). Where is the Love in Counselling? *Therapy Today, 28*(1), www.bacp.co.uk/bacp-journals/therapy-today/2017/december-2017/where-is-the-love-in-counselling (accessed 21 February 2021).

Owen, M. M. (2018). *I and Thou*. https://aeon.co/essays/all-real-living-is-meeting-the-sacred-love-of-martin-buber (accessed 21 February 2021).
Shohet, R. & Shohet, J. (2020). *In Love with Supervision*. Monmouth: PCCS Books.
Stolorow, R.D., & Atwood, G.E. (1992). *Contexts of Being: The Intersubjective Foundations of Psychological Life*. New York: Analytic Press.
Woods, S. L. (2009). Teaching Professionals Mindfulness. In F. Didonna (ed.), *Clinical Handbook of Mindfulness*. New York: Springer, pp. 463–75.

Chapter 6

Personal and professional development for relational practice

Introduction

Are we creating the best content and conditions for learning to develop the capacity to be relational practitioners? Are we reflecting on and seeking out the learning experiences that we need to develop the meta skills that enable us to engage in emergent dialogues with one another in supervision?

This chapter is my response to these questions. I explore the implications for those who are learning and those who teach them across the spectrum of initial and post-professional levels. I focus on the continuing professional development implications of our post hoc analysis in Chapter 5 and explore topics that include ways of knowing, ways of being, ways of learning and understanding, kinds of knowledge, and the challenges involved in integrating experiential relational practice into learning processes.

I propose a radical reformulation of the content and process of relational learning for relational practice, in groups and one to one, that is transformational for both learners and those facilitating their development. The approach to supervision learning and development described here is an evolutionary one: a mindfulness-based and compassionately co-created learning partnership that creates the conditions for emergence. Emergent learning supports the development of conscious awareness at all levels of mind, body, and spirit.

Being learners in a supervision relationship

When Jane and I met face to face for the first time, we were both beginners – I (Fiona) in the early stages of my role as a coach

DOI: 10.4324/9781315161280-6

supervisor, and Jane new to supervision. As we sat together, I was conscious of wanting to be welcoming and engaging, mentioning my qualifications and ideas I had about what supervision is. I was blissfully unaware that my anxiety was keeping me apart from Jane. On that day, we met one another with all our vulnerabilities and anxieties hidden from ourselves. Our implicit relational way of being in the world began to reveal itself to us during the next few months.

During phase two of our supervision relationship, Jane took the risk of sharing what she was feeling about our work together: that she felt incompetent. Her comments took me aback and I was touched by her honesty. I responded by sharing my own doubts about my competency. This reciprocal openness was the catalyst for change in our relationship.

Sitting with another person in a new supervision relationship, on a course, or in a workshop, we may find ourselves focusing on our need to give a good impression, to think of what to say next, perhaps feeling our need to fix their problems brought to us in a role-play, to offer answers, to be liked, and so on. Learning together and alone is an emotional business, as we cannot help but meet who we are as a person, sensing the ebbs and flows of our experience of being human. Some of what we are aware of will be conscious and some may well be expressed unconsciously, somatically through our body language, the tone of our speech, the rate of our breathing, and where our gaze falls.

Implications for continuing professional development

One of the foundational elements of preparation for relational practice is developing our capacity for meta-awareness, to awaken us to our developing self-knowledge – not only about *who* we are, but *how* we are, in the world of relationships, as well as how we make sense of events in our own lives.

We need to equip ourselves to become critically self-reflexive and curious about our day-to-day practice, what informs our ways of being and the knowledge on which we are drawing. Knowledge 'about' is never static: experience teaches us and builds our knowledge base. My concern is to enable us to be knowledgeable without over-identifying with our models and tools, but rather to be guided by what will serve the needs of the learning process in each moment. It means that relational learning begins with developing self-awareness, becoming conscious of how we have brought our ways of being in relationships learned as we became socialised in childhood. Deepening our knowledge of self, and especially how we engage relationally, is an ongoing process, a lifelong task should we be willing to accept it consciously.

In Chapter 3, we both described some of the lessons we have learned in life, discovering hitherto aspects of ourselves, which we are now able to apply to our practice. From being a person who loved analysing and seeking to understand the outer world, I have become free enough in myself to see that this way of being had cut me off from my feeling self, a protection developed to survive childhood difficulties. I now accept and enjoy being both an analytic thinker and a woman more at ease with her emotions, freer than ever to risk the ebbs and flows of personal and professional life, to learn relationally.

I am indebted to John Wilson, director at Temenos Education, for sending me a copy of the *Temenos Diploma in Person-Centred Counselling and Psychotherapy Trainee Handbook*. One of the final assessment criteria for this counselling course is that the student appears to be 'freely and deeply yourself', (Temenos Education, 2017–18: 17). I am led to wonder how much more delight in the learning process could be achieved if more of us felt free to be truly and deeply ourselves.

Being authentic in professional relationships

Our ways of being as course leaders and supervisors will naturally affect the relational experience of learners at all levels of education (Avenell, 2009; Brendgen, 2014). In her research on authenticity in relation to mindfulness teaching, Jane found that everything was taught through the person of the teacher – their way of being, their relational skills, and how they embodied what they were teaching. Martin Buber (quoted in Palmer, 1989: 16) considers that, 'All real living is meeting … and teaching is endless meeting.' Santorelli (1999: 97) describes the teacher–student relationship as 'an embodiment, a direct expression of interconnectedness and interdependence', where teaching is 'the vocation of becoming a true human being'.

In an article on relational education, Asheri (2015: 20) writes that authenticity 'is not straightforward but built on the shifting sands of multiple self-states in flux'. Surely the capacity to be authentic rests on learning to acknowledge and hold with compassion our fears and uncertainties about our competence and our vulnerability as human beings. Such learning can be and needs to be developed in the early stages of our professional development. When we are able to trust each other, and those who facilitate our learning, we can more easily accept our vulnerabilities with tenderness. This acceptance will enable us to take ourselves into relational work with compassion for our own humanity and that of others (Brendgen, 2014). We are then able to be true to the situations in which we find ourselves, noticing the ways of being called for by each situation (Bachkirova, 2020).

Authenticity thus asks much of us, as Ostaseski (2017: 130) writes:

> Authenticity requires trust in a deep inner wisdom and willingness to bring that wisdom into conscious action. Wisdom is not about age or expertise, tools, or roles.

I have a lot of tools that I have collected over the years, but I find that if I start pulling those tools out and setting them down between myself and my client, then one of us is sure to trip over them.

Ways of being and the key role of relational mindfulness

In our experience, relational mindfulness is the foundational meta skill of transformative relationships. It facilitates the capacity to be with what is, moment by moment. It also enables access to the relational field and empowers us to surrender the need for control.

Being present can become difficult when we feel threatened relationally – that is, when we are triggered into reactivity. Anxiety, fear, anger, shame, or any other stress-based emotion thus becomes something to explore, to be curious about, rather than hidden and interrupting the flow of giving and receiving in the dialogue. Relational mindfulness enables us to notice this and to then support each other, co-regulating our nervous systems.

In Chapter 4, we described how the practice of relational mindfulness supported us to connect with our subjective experience. We learned about our own ways of being in relationships by valuing knowledge derived from our practical experience, noticing how we were being with each other.

Those of us with much experience can be blind to what is happening relationally in each moment. In our work, relational mindfulness enabled us to learn together, to develop a way of being that was relationally conscious. For example, in the case study I describe that at the very early stage of our relationship when I was, as my supervisor so aptly put it, 'parading my wares', I was actually hiding my uncertainties. Gradually, my anxieties became extremely obvious to me as I tuned in to the effect they were having on my body (Aquilina, 2017).

Learning environment

It is imperative that all of us – trainers and supervisors alike – attend to our own ways of being, creating a climate of psychological safety so learners feel secure enough to receive and use the feedback for our development during experiential learning, (Edmondson, 2014). The same must be said about feedback from course members to one another, to learn to give feedback in a way that enhances the learning. Those who facilitate coaching and supervision courses and workshops find that students may be afraid to use themselves in their work – perhaps not yet ready to acknowledge that who they are and how they are being affects how they engage with their clients. They may even have an unhelpful mental image of the practitioner – perhaps as an expert who is there to work with models and tools where their humanness is bracketed out of the process. This view reflects an outdated concept of professional behaviour that sees professionals solely as having all the answers.

Making practice choices

What part of ourselves makes choices about how to practise as a coach and supervisor, and what other factors underpin decision-making? How we make sense of and draw from different theories is a complex mix. It includes who we are as an individual, our frames of reference, our values and beliefs, how we feel on the day, and what is evoked by each relational encounter (Cavicchia and Gilbert, 2018). Our responses are also a reflection of our social and emotional stage of development, which shapes how we make meaning and how we see our place in the world (Kegan, 1995).

We all have blind spots or unconscious biases that are likely to be incompatible with our espoused values. Feedback will support us to recognise that choosing a certain course of action at any moment is inevitably both a conscious and an unconscious act. In an exploratory study, Bachkirova's (2011) subjects reported that they were aware of being open to self-deception, and that it was part of being human. When we are enabled to become open to change, we develop and learn from feedback as a key part of becoming self-aware during basic training, followed by continuing personal and professional development and supervision

Self as instrument

Self as instrument is a widely referenced idea in the literature on coaching, supervision, and therapy (Aquilina, 2017; Bachkirova, 2011, 2016; Hawkins and McMahon, 2020; Hargaden, 2015; Silsbee, 2008). In many fields of practice, the quality of the relationship between client and practitioner has been found to be closely connected to the most effective work, whatever theoretical approach is applied (Wampold, 2001). Educating coaches and supervisors within this paradigm is therefore about developing the self of the coach as an instrument.

Learners who are fearful of using themselves as instruments need support and evidence that *who they are* and *how they are being relationally* are as important as the knowledge, models, and tools from which they may draw (Wampold, 2001). The aim must be for them to discover ways in which they can contribute and engage as fellow human beings with their clients' personal and professional developmental learning and performance needs.

So many of us are drawn to help others and, while being a good motivation, this desire has a shadow self. For example, you have met 'Helpful Harriet', my sub-personality – the compulsive helper trait. I was unaware of carrying her in my personality and so unable to acknowledge this aspect of my behaviour. I have learned to notice that Harriet arrives when I feel stuck during a session. I now introduce her to supervisees so we can both look out for her.

Clients working with an unaware professional could be disempowered from finding their own inner resources, and perhaps afraid to develop their own thinking and discover new ways of being. Central to my argument in this chapter is the idea that in a relational approach to coaching and supervision, practitioners need to bring an awareness of themselves as unique human beings, with their various traits, into their work with their clients. Operating with such self-awareness enables them to bring their way of being, their vulnerability, values, life experiences, approaches, and philosophies into how they engage in the relational field. The key here is to know and to feel compassion for the sum of who we are.

There are many paths to discovering what qualities of the self we each bring to our professional and personal lives. For example, the Coaching Signatures Profile (CSP) (Stevens, 2014), which was derived from Walker's (2009) Human Ecology Theory, suggests that we view our life as an ecological system. Unlike many psychometric tools, the CSP is based on the creation of an inner visual landscape, a metaphor for the coach's mental construct or way of being in their professional life. The CSP generates eight different coaching styles and measures the emergent relational space between the coach and coachee. It is evaluative and self-reflective, and gives a snapshot of the signature style of the coach while they recall different clients. The signature styles are also applicable to supervision practice. Learning our own signature style does not mean that our styles are set in stone. As we change and become socially and emotionally mature, our style becomes more varied and adapts to the relational work we do (Clutterbuck, 2020).

Inner cast of mini-selves

Each relationship calls forth different aspects of who we are as a professional, from expert advice-giver to dialogue partner. Bachkirova's (2016) concept of the self as having many 'mini-selves' or self-states invites us to consider and notice what parts of our selves we bring to our professional encounters with others. What roles are we playing and how are we playing them? What are our intentions, and are we wedded to a certain way of acting whatever the context? Are we able to include our 'more modest sense of self' as a fellow human being into our cast of mini-selves as we work relationally?

A key question for all who design continuing professional development courses and workshops for both coaches and supervisors is how to incorporate approaches that facilitate the discovery of their own inner cast of mini-selves (Bachkirova, 2017). The next step is to be aware of when and how their different mini-selves reveal themselves in their work with clients and how some of these different inner selves may be affecting the progress of their work.

The developmental path that we and our clients are following reflects the approach we take to the change process (Bachkirova, 2011). Our dialogues with others become the crucibles for change throughout our adult lives when we are willing to engage and able to learn with and from others. This relational way of being becomes not only aspirational but possible when, as supervisors, coaches, and educators, we are supported to set aside the fear-based drives of our own ego and our own desires for a particular outcome, and truly enter a relational space with no predetermined agenda. In adult development terms, this means we have become post-conventional or self-authoring (Kegan, 1995). This is the stage of our lives when we can instead be there in service as a 'dialogue guide' (Stelter, 2019) with our dialogue partner in an open-hearted and compassionate way.

Kinds of knowledge and experience

Learning from research

Kenneth Gergen (2015) makes the case for knowledge from research that is 'future forming', where it represents 'a shift from conception of knowledge as an individual possession into knowledge inhering within relations among people'. His approach is based on our having enough propositional knowledge to enable us to act thoughtfully. We may then become able to be improvisational when we find ourselves facing uncertainty and ambiguity. Here there is a mutual engagement in learning 'how to go on' together, a process that Shotter (2010) calls 'withness-thinking'. This approach is not unlike skilled jazz musicians, who have sufficiently mastered the basics of music-making to engage with band members from positions both of responding and leading as they play together, improvising as they go – artistry in motion.

Scholar practitioners, such as Alison Hodge (2014), who has been willing to explore her own and others' practice in the field of supervision, are rare. More of us could be supported and encouraged to inquire into our own practice when we feel inspired, as Jane and I have been to write this book. Few supervisors and coaches have the confidence to begin writing even short articles without support, let alone begin doctoral or master's studies, or write papers for peer reviewed journals.

Building the capacity for emotional regulation in relationship

We are, paradoxically, both unique individuals and interdependent human beings shaped relationally as we continue to grow, and to know ourselves in mind, body, and spirit. As social beings, we need to recognise that we are also playing a part in shaping others for good or ill, a responsibility for professionals who work relationally (Dana, 2018). We all need ways of learning that facilitate relational skills, and particularly those that help us develop the capacity to respond in moments that may trigger anxiety by allowing us to become sufficiently resilient to recover a steady state of readiness to continue. Triggers that arouse our anxiety can and do occur in all relationships, as well as in learning, teaching, and professional practice. It is a myth that any of us are untroubled at some level, so even the most resilient of us can be suddenly thrown off balance by sensing a threat to our self-esteem.

The capacity to stay steady in the ebbs and flows of the emotional demands of human relationships is known as being able to emotionally regulate. It means the capacity to be fully in the flow of being in relationships, able to deal with the emotional impact of the moment. We may not have learned this during our early attachment experiences. Recent research has shown that an individual's motivation and choice to engage their emotional regulation capacity, whether consciously or not, are frequently affected by the norms and beliefs of their own group or tribe (Porat et al., 2020). Group emotional norms are likely to be adopted when individuals feel the need to be identified as group members. This means that individuals who feel anxious and stressed by the felt need to conform may unconsciously sense that they must suppress their emotional needs. An individual who feels out of step with the group and considers leaving is more likely to be drawing on their own emotional regulation capacity. This finding has implications for all of us as we take part in learning and development groups of all kinds. A post-conventional frame of mind is more likely to provide considerable protection from 'group think', as at this stage our minds are free from conventional modes of thinking and from fears of diverging from social norms of behaviour.

The capability for emotional self-regulation is the responsibility of all educators and learners alike, to enable the co-creation of psychological safety, trust, and respect that facilitates mutual transformational learning, which can then extend out into professional practice.

Developing compassionate groupwork meta skills

Apart from being used widely in adult learning contexts at all levels, working with groups is becoming common in supervision. Faculty at the University of Hertfordshire have developed an interdepartmental course that prepares students to be compassionate in their behaviour towards their fellow students in group discussions. They learn together to co-create better conditions for learning and developing self-esteem, which are not based on being better than others, but rather performing well in a climate of self and other support (Gilbert, 2018). As part of their induction, new lecturers also do this course. Understanding group dynamics and group development is an essential part of the course. I believe courses such as this offer those new to group learning a way to become relationally conscious and to act with compassion towards others in their group.

Challenges involved in integrating experiential relational practice into courses and workshops

Many relationally challenging situations are likely to arise for coaches and supervisors during CPD. We may be challenged about our thinking, and for some of us this may affect who we believe ourselves to be. We need to become responsively adept during such challenging moments. The necessary mindfulness-based meta skills that enable us to respond rather than simply to react in challenging moments can be learned. The meta skill we most need in such moments is to be able to notice our reactivity and respond reflexively.

In the corporate world, relationships between leaders and those they manage are complex and often emotionally dysregulating (Reitz, 2015). Speaking truth to power is a relational action, and many employees are fearful of the response they may get when doing so. Fear of speaking up inevitably also arises in educational contexts that contain potentially conflictual power relationships, particularly those involving the assessment process and in making choices about the content and process of courses. Godward's (2019) literature survey on the topic of tutor–student conflicts on counselling courses identified six factors that led to such conflicts: personal issues and vulnerabilities of both student and trainer/educator; problematic interpersonal dynamics that may reflect projections of unresolved family dynamics; the unmet need for safety and trust in trainees; unacknowledged difficulties with power relationships; role conflict and ambiguity and transference and counter-transference issues. Further evidence is provided by Nelson et al. (2008).

During professional development courses and workshops, facilitators may misuse their power over those who challenge them. Fellow students may be critical of their peers about their behaviour in personal development groups. I was shocked to hear about one such incident from a supervisee and to recognise that some of the factors found by Godward (2019) were operating in this situation.

In this case, the student realised that, despite his own efforts to address the difficulties he was experiencing with the way tutors on his university counselling course conducted themselves in groups, staff were neither willing nor able to resolve his concerns. He felt he had been scapegoated by them as a troublemaker, and that as group facilitators, they had made no attempt to explore the dynamics operating among some students in the group meetings. He felt he had no choice but to make a formal complaint to the institution concerned.

As I reflected on this incident, which must have been deeply unsettling and difficult for all concerned, I recognised the vulnerability of the faculty members in that they appeared to lack both groupwork skills and emotional self-regulation capacity. Our vulnerability as human beings can be hard to bear, particularly when we are caught up in conflict situations. It is very likely that the tutors concerned were triggered into their survival behaviours and unable to access an emotionally regulated response. It seems that defensiveness and an abuse of power were the only responses available to them at the time. Given the ubiquity of varying degrees of childhood trauma, many of us will have developed anxious and insecure attachment styles, and this will certainly impact our capacity to stay steady and recover our equilibrium in the face of criticism from students, colleagues, and clients.

In this situation, the tutors were unable to stand back sufficiently to see the incidents as opportunities to approach students with an intention to work together compassionately to resolve their concerns. As a supervision course trainer, Robin Shohet gives a very moving account of his experience of being criticised by the student group (Shohet and Shohet, 2020). He describes the process that he facilitated, which helped to repair their relationship with him. The level of self-awareness and willingness to take the next courageous step towards a restoration process came from Shohet's willingness to see learning as a co-created process. He was prepared to model his vulnerability and his compassion for his students, and to show how to work with challenges that could otherwise have derailed the whole programme.

The example cited above demonstrates that there is a need for facilitators/educators to model relational meta skills, providing the skills, space, and time to work through interpersonal challenges from the outset. Relational practitioners can then start at the beginning of their training to learn experientially about who they are and how they are in relationships. This will support the building of the core meta skills of self-regulation and the capacity to stay steady in the face of emotionally challenging moments. These are requisite skills for all professionals working relationally (Dana, 2018). As learners experience being in the presence of educators who are relating with compassion and able to use their authority with ease, grace, and confidence, this will support their capacity to embody these qualities for themselves.

In her thesis on management education and on learning being the pathway to transformation of identity, Aram (2001) concludes that education is both a group and a social process, and thus an 'emotional business' for all concerned. She proposes a shift from thinking about education as a system to focusing on education in which 'students and teachers are both forming the process and being formed by it'. Aram further suggests that courses that take a traditional approach to teaching and learning 'actually damp down the potential for transformation and focus on maintaining the continuity in terms of the transmission of knowledge'. Here Aram is describing the difference between training as the transmission of knowledge and skills and education as a transformational experience for all parties towards new ways of being and acting.

Innovations in cross-domain professional development

There is a growing body of research on the value and efficacy of relational approaches to coaching and supervision (Cavicchia and Gilbert, 2018; De Haan, 2008, 2012; Hodge, 2014). Is it time to begin to redefine the boundaries or silos that keep each of us in our related practices of coaching, supervision, mentoring, and organisational consultancy as each of these practices requires relational meta skills that are foundational in each domain? Cross-professional courses bring each of the different practitioners to learn relational meta skills together. Providing experiential opportunities to learn these meta skills brings a challenge to loosen the ties that direct the focus of educators and professionals on 'getting it right' in terms of defining how our work is labelled as: 'Is this coaching? Is this mentoring? Is this supervision? Is this therapy?' Is the search for boundary maintenance and professionalisation in each domain stifling our thinking about what now needs to evolve in terms of how we educate for relational work? How do we prepare practitioners in ways that will enable them to become relationally and creatively adaptive, whatever the context of their practice?

Conclusion

There are many different approaches to teaching, evaluating, and learning relational practice. At the heart of all of them we find a process and a philosophy that can bring teachers and learners into partnership to co-create the core conditions for developing authentic and relationally skilled human beings. We need practitioners who can bring themselves fully and deeply into all their professional and personal dialogues. A relational learning and teaching perspective challenges us to design professional development in new ways that will engage all participants to collaborate in the learning process, including evaluation and knowledge creation.

We can see that the future growth of coaching and supervision depends on our being willing to respond to the challenge to change our ways of being. How far are we *all* willing to join collaboratively to develop our capacity to relate authentically, to transform our sense of self, and to find ways that are safe for the learning and discovery that are needed? The implications of our challenge for educators and trainers, as well as supervisors and coaches, require a radical reframing of both the content and process of courses, and the many forms of continuing personal and professional development. We cannot escape the fact that, in teaching and learning relationships, we will encounter our emotions as well as our ideas. Those of us engaged in pre- and post-professional teaching and learning have the potential and opportunity to engage in reciprocal transformational change.

A foundational aim of relational education is to enable us to become resilient enough to face the uncertainties and emotional challenges that we as supervisors, educators, and learners alike inevitably meet at work and in our personal lives, enabling us to develop and sustain all our relationships with ease, grace, and love. This aim can be realised by the adoption of a contemplative relational pedagogy, paving the way towards co-created teaching, evaluation, and learning (Gill and Gergen, 2020).

Summary

In this chapter, I (Fiona) have proposed a radical reframing of both the content and the processes that facilitate relational learning for relational practice and addressed the personal and interpersonal implications for all concerned. The chapter acknowledged that teaching and learning are emotionally challenging. I argued that relational mindfulness facilitates a climate of psychological safety in which all can be supported to engage with whatever arises in the ebb and flow of the relational field. I advocated learning in partnership that supports the development of compassion for all of who we are.

Questions for reflection

1 How important is relational learning in your development as a supervisor?
2 What kinds of research findings do you draw on to inform how you practise?
3 If you had the opportunity to co-create a course or workshop for supervisors, what would you bring to the design conversation?
4 What do you think about designing specific courses on relational meta skills for a range of those engaged in relational work, besides supervisors and coaches?

References

Aram, E. (2001). The Experience of Complexity: Learning as the Potential Transformation of Identity. PhD thesis, University of Hertfordshire.

Aram, E. (2015) Does Love Matter? Fear and Compassion in Organizations and Leadership. Lunchtime talk at the Tavistock Institute of Human Relations, London.

Aquilina, E. (2017). *Embodying Authenticity: A Somatic Path to Transforming Self, Team and Organisation*. Brighton: Live It.

Asheri, S., Carrol, R., Morrow, I. and Yellin, J. (2015). 'Still Evolving …': Reflections on Teaching Relational Psychotherapy. An Edited Summary of Their Conversation. *The Psychotherapist, 61*, 18–20. https://issuu.com/ukcp-publications/docs/61_the_psychotherapist_autumn_2015 (accessed 20 February 2021).

Avenell, K. (2009). Keys to Leadership: The Importance of Relational Pedagogy. *Australian Educational Leader, 31*(2), 31–2.

Bachkirova, T. (2011). *Developmental Coaching: Working with the Self*. Maidenhead: Open University Press.

Bachkirova, T. (2016). The Self of the Coach: Conceptualization Issues, and Opportunities for Practitioner Development. *Consulting Psychology Journal: Practice and Research, 68*(2), 143–56.

Bachkirova, T. (2020). Authenticity: How Do We Really Keep It Real? *Coaching at Work, 3*, 12–13.

Bachkirova, T., Jackson, P., Gannon, J., Iordanou, I. and Myers, A. C. (2017). Re-Conceptualising Coach Education from the Perspective of Pragmatism and Constructivism. *Philosophy of Coaching, 2*(2), 29–50.

Bachkirova, T. and Lawton Smith, C. (2015). From Competencies to Capabilities in the Assessment and Accreditation of Coaches. *International Journal of Evidence Based Coaching and Mentoring, 13*(2), 123–40.

Brendgen, J. (2014). Embodied Presence: A Heuristic Inquiry into Mindfulness Teachers' Experiences of Authenticity. MA thesis, University of Bangor.

Cavicchia, S. and Gilbert, M. (2018). *Theory and Practice of Relational Coaching*. London: Routledge.

Clutterbuck, D. (2020). *The Leader's Guide to Being Coached: A Practical Guide* (2nd ed.). Liverpool: Wordscape.

Clutterbuck, D. and Megginson, D. (2011). Coach Maturity: An Emerging Concept. In L. Wildflower and D. Brennan (eds), *The Handbook of Knowledge-Based Coaching: From Theory to Practice*. Chichester: John Wiley & Sons.

Dana, D. (2018). *The Polyvagal Theory in Therapy: Engaging the Rhythm of Regulation*. New York: W. W. Norton.

De Haan, E. (2008). *Relational Coaching: Journeys Towards Mastering One-to-One Learning*. Chichester: John Wiley & Sons.

De Haan, E. (2012). *Supervision in Action: A Relational Approach to Coaching and Consulting Supervision*. New York: McGraw Hill.

Edmondson, A. (2014). Psychological Safety: The History, Renaissance, and Future of an Interpersonal Construct. *Annual Review of Organizational Psychology and Organizational Behaviour, 1*, 23–43.

Gergen, K. L. (2015). From Mirroring to World-Making: Research as Future Forming. *Journal for the Theory of Social Behaviour, 45*(3), 287–310.

Gergen, K. L. and Dixon-Roman, E. J. (2014). Social Epistemology and the Pragmatics of Assessment. *Teachers College Record, 116*(11), 1–22.

Gilbert. T., Doolan, M., Beka, S., Spencer, N., Crotta, M., and Davari, S. (2018). Compassion on University Degree Programmes at a UK University: The Neuroscience of Effective Group Work. *Journal of Research in Innovative Teaching & Learning, 11*(1). www.emerald.com/insight/content/doi/10.1108/JRIT-09-2017-0020/full/pdf?title=compassion-on-university-degree-programmes-at-a-uk-university-the-neuroscience-of-effective-group-work (accessed 20 February 2021).

Gill, S. and Gergen, K. J. (2020). Education Evaluation: A Relational Perspective. In S. McNamee, M. M. Gergen, C. Camargo-Borges, and E. F. Rasera (eds), *The Sage Handbook of Social Constructionist Practices*. Thousand Oaks, CA: Sage, pp. 402–12.

Godward, J. (2014). Student–Tutor Conflict in Counsellor Training. *Therapy Today, 25*(8), 18–21.

Godward, J. (2019). Conflict and Difficulties in Personal Development Groups. In J. Godward, H. Dale, and C. Smith (eds), *Personal Development Groups for Trainee Counsellors*. London: Routledge, pp. 71–82.

Hargaden, H. (ed.) (2015). *The Art of Relational Supervision, Clinical Implications of the Use of Self in Group Supervision*. London: Taylor and Francis.

Hawkins, P. and McMahon, A. (2020). *Supervision in the Helping Professions*. Maidenhead: Open University Press.

Hodge, A. (2014). *An Action Research Inquiry into What Goes on in Coaching Supervision to the End of Enhancing the Coaching Profession*. www.semanticscholar.org/paper/An-action-research-inquiry-into-what-goes-on-in-to-Hodge/01e0e8212e4eda6d44d053b77b675c881c90d3ba (accessed 20 February 2021).

Kegan, R. (1995). *In Over Our Heads: Mental Demands of Modern Life*. Cambridge, MA: Harvard University Press.

Nelson, M. L., Barnes, K. L., Evans, A. L., and Triggiano, P. J. (2008). Working with conflict in clinical supervision: Wise supervisors' perspectives. *Journal of Counselling Psychology, 55*(2), 172–84.

Ostaseski, F. (2017). *The Five Invitations*. London: Bluebird.

Palmer. P. (1989). *The Courage to Teach*. San Francisco: Jossey Bass.

Porat, R., Tamir, M., and Halperin, E. (2020). Group-Based Emotion Regulation: A Motivated Approach. *Emotion, 20*(1), 16–20.

Reitz, M. (2015). *Dialogue in Organizations: Developing Relational Leadership*. London: Palgrave Macmillan.

Silsbee, D. (2008). *Presence-Based Coaching: Cultivating Self-Generative Leaders Through Mind Body and Heart*. San Francisco: Jossey-Bass.

Santorelli, S. (1999). *Heal Thyself: Lessons in Mindfulness in Medicine*. Victoria, BC: Crown Publications.

Shohet, R. and Shohet J. (2020). *In Love with Supervision: Creating Transformative Conversations.* Monmouth: PCCS Books.

Shotter, J. (2010). *Social Construction on the Edge: 'Withness' Thinking and Embodiment.* Chagrin Falls, OH: Taos Institute.

Stelter, R. (2019). *The Art of Dialogue in Coaching Towards Transformative Exchange.* London: Routledge.

Stevens, P. (2014). *Coaching Signatures Profile.* https://supervision.uk.com (accessed 20 February 2021).

Temenos Education (2017) *Temenos Diploma in Person-Centred Counselling and Psychotherapy Trainee Handbook.* Sheffield: Temenos Education.

Walker, S. P. (2009). *A Brief Introduction to the Theory of Human Ecology.* London: Simon Walker.

Wampold, B. E. (2001). *The Great Psychotherapy Debate: Models, Methods and Findings.* Mahwah, NJ: Lawrence Erlbaum.

Chapter 7

Summary and conclusion

Introduction

Our experience reveals that coaches and supervisors need to develop foundational capacities both during and after their training. We propose an evolutionary model of relationally mindful education in coaching and supervision that regards the following meta skills as fundamental both in underpinning effective relational practice and in supporting us all to survive and thrive in an uncertain world:

- See ourselves as human beings first and as professionals second.
- Learn to accept our vulnerability and our humanity with tenderness. This will support us to become compassionate and open-hearted.
- Be reflexively conscious, self-aware, and aware of the relational field.
- Be open to emergence and not-knowing in a co-created dialogue.
- Be willing to engage in reciprocal learning.
- Be open to shifts in interpersonal perspective.
- Enhance our capacity for emotional self-regulation, which will help to develop resilience – the capacity to recover appropriately when challenged or triggered.
- Be open to somatic resonances – that is, being aware of implicit relational knowledge held in the body.
- Be supported to develop our gifts without fear of failure.
- Attend to and sustain ourselves through continuing personal and professional development.

DOI: 10.4324/9781315161280-7

The challenges for us as supervisors when seeking to either enter initial training or seek continuing professional development are to:

- Seek help when feeling overwhelmed by personal and professional challenges.
- Take seriously our own continuing need for self-care.
- Continue being in supervision and change to a different supervisor if the relationship does not meet our deepest learning needs.
- Engage in peer learning communities.
- Carry out scholar practitioner research at master's and doctoral level.
- Contribute to conferences with your experience, our own research findings, case studies and live demonstrations.
- Send our writing to a variety of magazines and academic journals.
- Be prepared to partner with training providers to co-create courses that we need at this stage in our development.

We regard this time in the history of our profession as an opportunity to take the next step in the evolution of our practice. We are calling on all of us – supervisors, educators, professional bodies and all practitioners in the helping professions – to undertake a major re-evaluation of our approach to professional and personal learning and development. We are calling for *a relational and contemplative pedagogy* so that we can learn together from an emerging future, which surely involves the most profound challenge of all: climate change (Barbezat and Bush, 2014). Now more than ever, we need models of education and continuing professional and personal development that will enable us all to continue to learn who we are becoming; to respond with grace, love, and wisdom to those with whom we work; and to keep in touch with emerging approaches to our practice and our responsibilities as citizens.

Reference

Barbezat, D. P. and Bush, M. (2014). *Contemplative Practices in Higher Education: Powerful Methods to Transform Teaching and Learning*. San Francisco: Jossey-Bass.

Appendix

Excerpt from our supervision agreement

This is an excerpt from our supervision agreement, which we explore with our clients at the onset of our work together. This took shape during the writing of our book.

Model of supervision

Because each supervisor has their own style, I thought it might be helpful for you to know how I like to work.

I take a mindfulness-based relational approach, which supports reciprocal learning and mutual transformation. This approach changes the quality of the supervisor–supervisee relationship and deepens our capacity to learn together.

In my experience, the conditions that support mutual transformational learning in supervision include:

- Creating a psychologically safe container for our work together. In support of this, the conversations that unfold in the sessions will be held in confidence.
- Offering opportunities to mindfully pause in the moment as a way to connect with the body, enhance self-awareness, and support a deeper reflection.
- My sharing that I may be feeling or sensing something in the field, either somatically or emotionally, and that we might use this information to deepen our inquiry.
- Working with silence as a support for clarity of reflection, generative thinking, and insight, and practising this important meta-skill as a way to strengthen client relationships.

- Learning to be comfortable with not knowing as a means to work more emergently. As we settle into being with what is here now with an attitude of curiosity, this can facilitate the opening up of new vistas of learning through reducing the sense of 'striving to do something to get somewhere'.
- Where relevant and appropriate, sharing our personal life experiences with the intention to contribute to the learning.
- Inviting mutual vulnerability and honesty, particularly in those moments where discomfort is felt by either or both of us.
- Recognising our common humanity, in that we are both learning from each other, we are both fallible and there is no 'getting things right' for either of us. In alignment with this, encouraging you to make choices aligned with your personal values in contrast to prescriptive ways of doing things.
- Requesting that you to raise any concerns you have related to your supervision with me in service of strengthening psychological safety, our working relationship, and optimising the conditions for our mutual learning.

Ways of learning

As your supervisor, I will be responsible for offering you, as best I can, the support you need to develop both horizontally and vertically – that is, focusing on your coaching skills enhancement as well as on your adult development. Here, within the context of your coaching practice, we can explore the personal capacities and meta skills that enhance our capacity to deal with volatility, uncertainty, complexity, and ambiguity.

Index

CPD abbreviation = continuing professional development